D1610739

Why Vegan
is the New Black

More than 100 delicious meat and dairy free meal ideas your whole family will love

Deborrah Cooper

Many of the designations used by manufacturers and sellers to distinguish their products are claimed as registered trademarks. When those designations appear in this book, and where we are aware of a copyright claim, those designations have been set out in initial caps and/or indicated by the registered symbol.

Why Vegan is the New Black
©2014 by Deborrah Cooper

Interior layout and design
Steven McClelland and Deborrah Cooper
Cover design Tarryn Cooper
Photography by Deborrah Cooper

ISBN: 978-0-9909713-8-2

Why Vegan is the New Black
www.whyveganisthenewblack.com

Why Vegan *is the* New **Black**

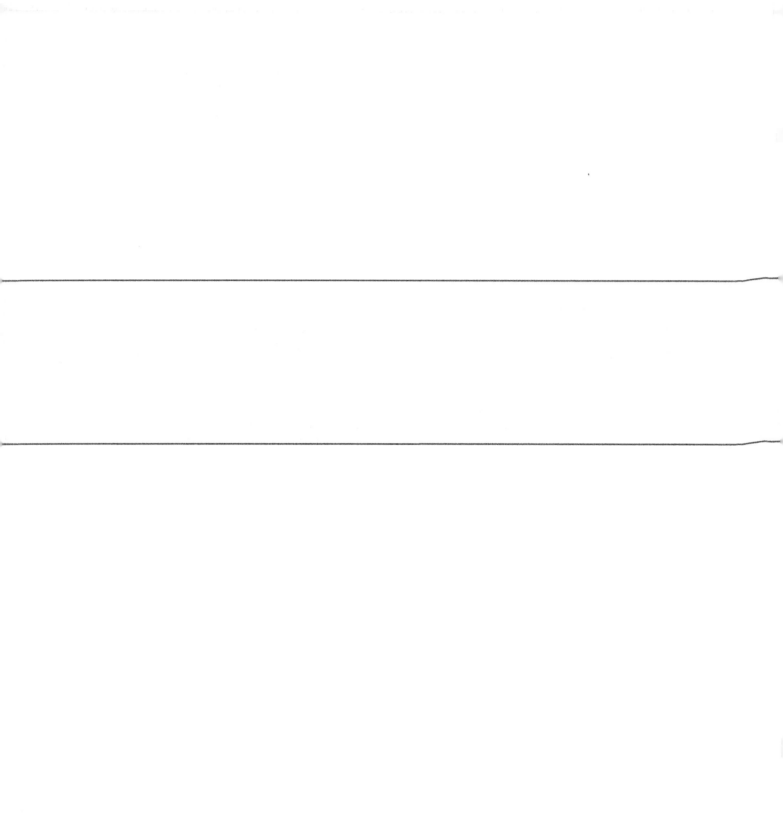

Contents

Why Vegan is the New Black

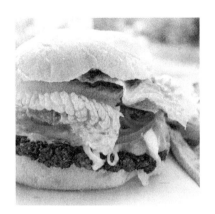 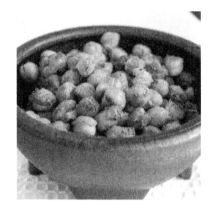 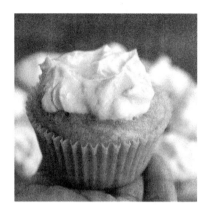

Introduction

The Long Journey to Vegan

My maternal great-great-great grandmother was born a slave. Despite her bleak beginnings in life, she lived to be 110 - still cooking, cleaning, gardening, walking for miles every day, and doing everything she wanted to do without medication or assistance. My paternal grandmother died in her 90s in very good health, living more than 60 years after being struck by lightening. My own mother is a lean and healthy senior, free of medication and leading a full, active life.

Okay, looking at my family tree, it's apparent that I come from a gene pool of hearty, healthy folks. Nutritionally I was off to a good start as well. I grew up eating home grown collard and mustard greens, carrots pulled fresh from the earth, freshly picked tomatoes, pinto and navy beans, black eyed peas, cornbread, and lots of home made soups and stews. We rarely went out to eat at restaurants, didn't have soda pop in the house, and I can almost remember the times we ate fast food burgers and chicken.

As a child, my life was also full of movement. In the era before video games took over, my brothers and I entertained ourselves by playing outside - skating, running, climbing, and riding our bikes for hours. I participated in team sports, and was involved in Girl Scouts as well. In my 20s, I jogged 4-5 miles several times per week, jumped rope, and took aerobic dance classes. In my 30s I became a serious gym rat and personal trainer, acquiring six national certifications in fitness, nutrition, senior fitness, and special populations (people with joint and other serious health problems).

In other words, I had the keys to unlock a long, full and healthy life well into my senior years. But I hit a few potholes on the road, and somewhere, somehow I got off track. The stresses of life took their toll, and my body began to show signs of deterioration.

The final "nail in the coffin" so to speak was a doctor visit to treat a problem with one of my feet. I was also suffering from serious gastrointestinal problems – stomach pains so severe I thought I was getting an ulcer. I was issued an immobilizer/walking "boot" for my foot which provided immediate relief. But since I hadn't been in for awhile my doctor insisted on a major blood panel.

When the blood work came back, I was in for a shock. Not only had I developed high blood pressure, I also had slightly elevated cholesterol, and blood sugar which put me in the category of prediabetic.

"How could that happen?" I asked myself incredulously? "Where had I gone wrong?" Especially since I KNEW the afflictions I was diagnosed with are linked to food intake, and are very preventable. Though I was shocked, confused, and felt pitiful, I had to be honest with myself and admit this situation was my doing, and completely my fault.

I wasn't exercising as I had been previously; but the most serious and detrimental change was my eating habits. Though I still cooked when I could find time, I'd slowly adopted the Standard American Diet (SAD) of high carb/low nutrient foods, mass manufactured on-the-go type foodstuffs. It was normal over the course of a week to have sugary muffins made with refined white flour, donuts, nachos and burritos with fattening cheese and sour cream, burgers and fries, barbecued ribs, cakes and pies, and rich buttery cream sauces and dressings.

Since I worked long hours, takeout Chinese, pizza, grocery store rotisserie chickens, and fast-cooking frozen or packaged side dishes became standard dinner fare. Cold cuts and deli sandwiches, taqueria tacos, and breakfast sandwiches rounded out my meals.

For more than two years I'd failed to do much of anything to maintain the health and fitness I'd worked so hard to achieve. My body was clearly showing the results of that neglect, as I'd gained more than 20 pounds and was faced with the possibility of some serious chronic diseases.

After our consultation, my doctor called in three prescriptions – two for hypertension and one for acid reflux. She also shared some sage advice: "you need to do something about this situation, and you need to do it now."

Hey, what can I say? There's something about staring at a blood work printout with anything outside the range of normal in bright red that gets your attention. You can't avoid the fact that you're in a bad spot. And every time I looked at those lab results I wanted to kick myself.

I'd taken decades of excellent health for granted, and ignored the fact I was not 21 anymore. It was a real wake up call. I had to accept that it was time to make some changes to my lifestyle, and I needed to make them immediately.

Determined to get my health and body back, I started a light fitness program. Wearing that heavy, bulky immobilizing boot on my foot made exercise awkward and exhausting, but I was able to do some standing and sitting work with dumbbells, a large fitness ball, and stretch bands.

I also pored through my fitness books and dozens of medically-related websites, refreshing myself on the fundamentals of nutrition and disease processes, and reviewed more up-to-date research on human health. From everything I read, it seemed the fastest, most long-lasting and impressive results were achieved by those who switched to a plant based diet.

So that's what I did.

My first task was to go through all the cabinets and the refrigerator with a fine-toothed comb. I gave or threw away ANYTHING that would not fit my new eating plan, or help me achieve my health goals. All bakery items, butter, eggs, cheese, crackers, packaged convenience foods, , fish, and poultry, bacon, canned chili and soups, canned milks, lunch meat, etc. All gone.

The second thing I did was tell my doctor I was going to adopt a plant based diet and become a vegan. Since she's been my doctor for 15 years, she felt quite comfortable bluntly asking me "do you know what the hell you're doing? I'm sending you to a dietitian!"

The appointment with the dietitian was informational. However, the standard protocol for treatment of pre-diabetics at my medical center is that of The American Diabetic Association (ADA). According to everything I'd read recently, published by leaders in treatment of diabetes with diet, there were far more effective treatments available. Dr. Neal Barnard, Dr. Joel Fuhrman, Dr. Caldwell Esselstyn, Dr. John McDougall and Dr. T. Colin Campbell were getting amazing results lowering blood sugar on a plant based diet at speeds which eclipsed those of the ADA.

The first few weeks were rough, as I eased into my dietary change by eating a lot of salads and sucking down smoothies. I half-heartedly counted my carb intake, but found it tedious and stressful, so I switched to the plant based diet and ignored carb counting. I diligently logged my food online however, then printed out my daily sheets and took them with me to my follow up visit. I was happy to see that in just six weeks I'd lost eight pounds without even trying!

I discussed my plant centered meal plan with the dietitian during my follow-up visit, and found her extremely positive about the changes I was making. I left the dietitian's office feeling like I was finally back on track.

However, since woman cannot live on salads and smoothies alone, I had to get more comfortable cooking new foods. The Mad Scientist in me enjoys making concoctions, potions, and mixes of all kinds. I turned that interest towards creating dishes that would make my vegan journey not only healthful, but tasty. The foundation for *Why Vegan is the New Black* was laid.

Does that sound like everything was smooth as silk and we all lived happily ever after? If only! Maybe I was naive, but I really believed family and friends would be more focused on the health issues I was attempting to correct than they were the fact that I gave up meat, eggs and dairy.

Instead, I was broadsided by unexpected criticism, and told that a vegan diet was "unnecessary" and "ridiculous," especially for an African American.

"Everybody needs to eat meat! Where are you gonna get your protein from?"

"What? You grew up eating meat and eggs and all that...what's the difference now?"

"I swear, you Californians. Why can't you just eat regular food like everybody else?"

"That's part of your heritage. Your people are southerners, and southerners eat ham, eggs, beef brisket, and ribs. What are you trying to prove?"

"Oh, so you're gonna be one of those freaky weird hippie vegans, huh?"

Sigh. I have to admit—vegans and vegetarians have gotten a bad rap. For decades people would roll their eyes at the mention of someone being vegan, picturing some wheat grass drinking, alfalfa sprout eating, carrot juicing, animal rights activisting, long haired freak. I have to admit that I was, at one time, one of them.

In reality, veganism has gone mainstream and is gaining in popularity every year. As a matter of fact, a study commissioned by the Vegetarian Resource Group in 2010 reports that approximately five percent of the U.S. population is vegetarian (close to 16 million people), and about half of those are vegan. With a nationwide population estimated to be 313.9 million according to the 2012 Census, eight million people may seem like a drop in the bucket. The key point here is that the number of vegans in the U.S. has doubled since 2009, so I'm obviously not the only one who made this choice. Moreover, 79% of those who chose to go vegan are women – just like me.

The study also revealed that about a third of Americans are eating vegan or vegetarian meals more often, though they don't officially declare themselves to be either. The growing popularity of Meatless Monday (www. meatlessmonday.com) in schools and homes means that more than 100 million people, or just under one-third of the U.S. population, is opting to eat a plant based diet at least some of the time.

There are half a dozen different designations for people who have or are in the process of reducing their dependence on animal products, but here are the four most common:

Vegan - Does not eat meat, poultry, fish, dairy, eggs or honey

Vegetarian - Does not eat meat, poultry or fish

Pescetarian - Eats fish/shellfish occasionally, but no meat or poultry

Meat Reducers - Working on eating less meat for ethical or environmental reasons; may participate in Meatless Monday.

I'm excited about these changes in dietary trends due to several important factors:

(1) American Adults Are Fat. It is reported that more than one-third (78.6 million) of American adults are obese. (To qualify as obese your body weight must be 20% or greater than what it should be.) Obesity is reported to be greatest amongst African Americans (with 47.8% of the population falling into the obese category), followed by Hispanics (42.5%), non-Hispanic whites (32.6%), and non-Hispanic Asians (at 10.8%). Obesity is also greater in the middle-aged demographic (40-59 years of age), with 39.5% of us eating too much of the wrong foods and not getting enough exercise.

(2) Childhood Obesity. Since children eat what their parents eat, poor diets and obesity tend to be generational. Though obesity rates amongst small children aged 2-5 have declined by 43% according to a 2014 report by The Centers for Disease Control, one-third of American children are still considered to be overweight or obese. Among American children aged 6–11, obesity increased from 7% in 1980 to nearly 18% in 2012. And for adolescents and teens 12–19 years old, the number of obese children increased 320%, going from 5% to nearly 21% of children over the same period. Overweight children are often teased, bullied and rejected socially by their peers. A nation full of overweight and obese children means our babies are also at increased risk for heart disease, diabetes, and strokes in adulthood. (www.cdc.gov/healthyyouth/obesity/facts.htm)

(3) We Eat an Amazing Amount of Meat and Cheese. Americans eat almost twice the amount of meat recommended by the USDA. That may not seem like a big deal if you're into eating a lot of protein, but consider this: In 1909 the average American consumed just 124 pounds of meat, and less than one pound of cheese per year. However, by the year 2000 that number had increased to more than 200 pounds of animal flesh, and more than 33 pounds of cheese annually. The majority of the meat and cheese ingested in the USA is processed through huge plants. Many health professionals and consumers have valid concerns about the process of killing and butchering the animals, as well as cloning, often fatal bacterial outbreaks (Staphylococcus aureus, E.Coli, Listeria, salmonella and Campylobacter), growth hormones and antibiotic use, meat recalls, and spotty plant inspections.

(4) Our Health is Taking a Hit. Many debilitating diseases are linked to food intake and weight, such as Type 2 diabetes, Alzheimer's, heart disease, certain cancers, hypertension, and strokes. Coupled with the joint pain of osteoarthritis, elevated blood lipids, sleep apnea, asthma, and gallstones, you can see that getting your weight under control so you can enjoy a medication-free life is important. Americans have a lot of

other problematic afflictions related to diets low in fiber and high in fat like constipation, hemorrhoids, diverticulitis and colon cancer. Experts recommend that we get 14 grams of dietary fiber for every 1000 calories consumed. Yet, the average American eating the SAD diet of animal and diary products, processed carbohydrates, fat, and sugar is lucky to get 12 grams over the course of an entire day.

Changing my diet did wonders for me, and I'm convinced it is a path you should investigate. A delicious and varied plant-centered diet helped me drop undesirable body fat and pounds without trying. Changing how I ate also helped me get my blood sugar and blood pressure under control, thereby reducing risks of coronary heart disease and stroke by half *in just eight weeks.*

I've openly shared information about my health problems and journey back to wellness because I think it's important for you to know the power food has to heal. I was my own guinea pig in this endeavor, which means I am a living, breathing, testimonial to the almost magical changes that can be achieved by eliminating animal-based foods from your diet. I am living proof that eradicating processed, packaged "instant," "quick," or processed foods can make you feel better, look far younger than your years, feel more energetic, and drop pounds/inches effortlessly.

It was important... no mandatory, that my meals taste good, have an enticing aroma, beautiful color, and that they be just as satisfying as meals created with animal products. I'm sure you expect nothing less. *Why Vegan is the New Black* was produced to support those who are hesitating (but curious about veganism), to take the leap and give it a try.

Within these pages are fabulous recipes for classic American, southern, Cajun and soul food dishes that you and your family are probably already familiar with. I understand that many readers aren't comfortable in the kitchen. It's important for your health that you cook your own food, because you'll always know exactly what you are eating. Cooking at home will also allow you to create and share family traditions handed down through generations. Home cooking is much less expensive than eating out or picking up food all the time, so you'll save a quite a lot of money.

The ability to cook is an essential life skill, something everyone can and should learn how to do. I've taken great pains to lead you step-by-step, fully explaining each process and how to do it. You'll be delighted by vegan versions of buttermilk pancakes, lasagna, spicy tacos, juicy burgers, spaghetti & meatballs, red beans and rice with andouille sausage, buffalo wings, fluffy biscuits, chicken fried steak and gravy, tuna salad, and even fried chicken.

Maybe it all sounds good, but you're confused about how to get started with the transition from meat-eater to plant-eater? Don't worry! With this cookbook in hand, you'll soon discover that plant based meals can be just as delectable, just as visually appealing, and just as satisfying to every member of your household as meals created with animal products.

Why Vegan is the New Black will inspire you to cook at home by providing dozens of ways to vary and improve your diet. You'll be motivated to include more nutritious fresh fruits, beans, greens and other vegetables, and whole grains in your diet than you've probably ever eaten before.

I have a few suggestions that will make things easier for you:

#1 As you move through this book you'll see ingredients that are vegan staples, but which you might be unfamiliar – nutritional yeast, liquid aminos, kombu seaweed, tofu, tahini, quinoa (pronounced "keen-wah"), chickpea flour, and agave ("ahh-gah-vay") are a few that are used frequently. My first suggestion is that you plan your menu for the day (or even the next 2-3 days), then journey to the farmer's market or produce stand to get the ingredients you need, if you don't already have them on hand.

#2 My second suggestion is that you invest in either a crock pot or a pressure cooker. For busy working parents, either of these appliances can be a life-saver. You'll be able to get a nutritious, home cooked meal on the table in 60 minutes or less from the time you walk in the door.

The growing popularity of plant based eating and veganism is setting new standards for American society. It's not enough to have a long life – people want to have a long and healthy life, fully capable of participating in the activities they've enjoyed for decades.

It is my hope that *Why Vegan is the New Black* will prove to you that becoming a vegan can be a wonderfully exciting adventure. Whether you plan to transition over a few months as you slowly remove meat and diary from your diet, or just want to eat a plant centered diet a few days per week, I got you. Your meals can be both easy to make and scrumptious.

Americans are sick and tired of being sick and tired, and are doing something about it by changing their nutrition. Focusing on improving our health by reducing or eliminating animal products from our diet has become the new normal.

And that's *Why Vegan is the New Black*.

Now let's get started!

Deborrah Cooper

Why Vegan is the New Black

More than 100 meat and dairy free meal ideas your whole family will love

Deborrah Cooper

Making The Transition

Though many people would like to modify their diet and take steps towards eating a plant based diet or becoming vegetarian/vegan, the number one stumbling block is not knowing how to start. There are several approaches you can take, which I believe are linked to your personality.

I like to use the analogy of going to the beach to explain the process, because it's something we can all relate to. As I view it, there are four ways for you to transition to a plant based diet, just as there are four types of beach-goers:

#1: The Sandcastle Builder. These are the individuals who lounge about on the sand. Their ice chest is within arm's reach, along with their suntan oil. They're at the beach primarily to play on the sand, and work on their tan. They enjoy watching others frolic and swim, but they don't really get IN the water themselves. They are frequently seen at the water's edge filling up a bucket or two with water, which they bring back to their area of the beach and use to construct a beautiful sandcastle. Some are more active, and will play beach volleyball or Frisbee. They may spend hours on these land-based endeavors, and never actually dip a single body part into the ocean.

The Sandcastle Builder makes a concerted effort to eat more fruits and vegetables, and may give up red meat while still eating chicken and fish. Some may have a meatless meal every now and then... like pancakes made with eggs and butter (leaving out the side of bacon or sausage); or a veggie burger with cheese along with fries and a shake. The Sandcastler is often referred to as "meat-reducers" and "pescetarians."

#2: The Wader/Splasher. These are the folks who approach the ocean with trepidation and often squeals. They'll jump and hop across the hot sand towards the ocean, but they keep going forward. Once at the water's edge, they stick one foot in to test the water temperature, then quickly pull it back out to determine if it's tolerable or not. You may observe them moments later kicking water as they walk or jog along the water's edge. After a few minutes of standing or walking along ankle deep water, they may walk out a little further, until the water is calf or knee level. They'll then bend forward and scoop water to splash their torso and thighs. However, their feet stay safely on land, and their hair never gets wet.

The Wader/Splasher approach to a vegan transition is quite meticulous and usually cautious. They'll do extended web research, read several books, watch educational videos, speak with their doctor, try vegan restaurants and vegan recipes. This type is usually drawn to Meatless Monday, No Meat for a Week, and those 21-day and 30-day vegan challenge programs. They seek the opportunity to "test the waters," but maintain an "out" with their feet safely on the land of the omnivore. If they do get in the water, it's usually with a paddle board or some sort of flotation device that helps keep their head above water; they feel safer that way. The Wader/Splasher can play in the ocean of veganism for as little as a few weeks to several years as they slowly phase out animal products, one at a time.

#3: The Walk Out Then Swim. These are the individuals who eye the water with a smile. They strip off their clothes and fold them neatly, then put on their sun block and goggles, and perhaps a rubber swim cap. They stride purposefully across the beach, directly to the water's edge. Without hesitation they walk straight out to chest height, then give themselves over to the ocean and start swimming. The joy and peace they feel is almost palpable as they swim, float, kick, turn flips and splash about. When they get back to land it's with a big smile and the certainty that they'll go back in the water in a bit, and if you want, you can join them.

The Walking Swimmer type prepares carefully for the transition to a plant based diet. They usually begin by adding more vegetables and fruits, then set a "start date" for the vegan eating plan to begin in earnest. Over a short period of time they eat all the animal products in their home without purchasing more; those that remain the day before start date are tossed out or given away. They get rid of anything that would tempt them. Their home is well stocked with staple food items, appliances, spices, and books needed to achieve their goals. They may be a bit cautious, but their mind is made up that this is the direction they're going to go. They are confident in their decision, so they let nothing deter them. Strong advocates of a vegan diet and lifestyle, they're patient and kind to others who seek knowledge and information. As a matter of fact, they're so positive, and make the change seem so enjoyable, that others are inspired to join them on their journey.

#4: THE FULL TILT. These are the people who make the decision to get into the water, and they do it! Immediately, without fear, without putting a toe in or wading or anything that shows hesitation. At the beach they're the ones you see throw down their stuff in a heap, then run across the sand and jump right into the water without a care about the temperature, their hair, or anything else. Their decision to jump in, once made, is irreversible. They want to get going on changing their life TODAY, not tomorrow.

The Full Tilt vegan goes "cold turkey" into veganism almost overnight. Sometimes the sudden change is precipitated by a medical diagnosis of a serious health condition for which dietary changes are the solution. However, most times the decision to become vegan is made by the Full Tilter immediately after learning shocking facts about the commercial meat production and dairy industries. Few people have the stomach to learn the ugly truths about animal cruelty in the name of food, and still desire to eat meat.

No matter which personality type you are, there are a few basic guidelines that will make the transition a much smoother one:

Stay Positive! Though they know conceptually that this is a great change to make, there are some people who spend a lot of time focusing on what they aren't "able to" eat anymore. My suggestion is to think about what you're gaining vs. what you're giving up. Life is all about deciding if the glass before you is half full, or half empty. So think of this dietary change as a positive step for your life, your body, and your planet. Instead of feeling deprived, you can feel empowered because you've taken charge of your health.

Read, Watch and Learn. Take the time to educate yourself on the many benefits of adopting a plant based lifestyle. There are literally hundreds of books and websites with excellent information on plant based diets, veganism and health. You can also find many free movies online that will be helpful; others are available with paid subscription services. A few of my favorites are *Vegucated*, *Food Inc.*, *Hungry for Change*, *Forks Over Knives*, *Super Size Me*, *May I Be Frank*, *Cowspiracy*, and *Earthlings*.

Set Yourself Up for Success. Create a menu plan for your first few days of vegan eating, then go out and purchase the items you'll need to make those meal dreams come true. Start stocking your kitchen with what you'll need to create a wide variety of meals (see Appendix B). Familiar foods will make things easier – oatmeal with chopped nuts, almond milk and an orange for breakfast, or a big salad with lots of chopped vegetables and chickpeas or kidney beans for lunch. Instead of hitting the nearest junk food restaurant after your workout, bring dried fruit and nuts, or a green smoothie made with pea protein powder, powdered greens and maca in your gym bag. Add water and shake, then drink.

Find Substitutions for Your Favorite Foods. Investigate plant based replacements for some of the things you like to eat most. Modern grocery and health food stores offer vegan and vegetarian foods in both the dairy and freezer sections. Though ideally, unprocessed natural state whole foods should comprise 75% of your diet, that's probably unrealistic and unnecessarily stressful for the transitioning vegan. If you like corn dogs, there are vegan alternatives. If you like meatballs with your spaghetti, there are vegan options available. If you like deli-style lunch meat sandwiches or pizza, there are plant based alternatives for those as well.

Commit Yourself to Change. Whether you opt to jump in Full Tilt style, eat vegan until 5:00 pm, eat vegan five days per week, or you drop animal products one at a time over a period of months, make a plan for yourself and stick to it. The road to success is traveled one step at a time. For the transitioning vegan that means taking things meal by meal, day by day.

Pay Attention to Your Gut. You may notice a change in bowel habits and experience bloating and gassiness in the early transition stage. That's because your body is not accustomed to processing so much fiber. If you experience digestive upset (flatulence, sudden diarrhea, or constipation), it might be best to slow down your transition process. Gradually increasing the amount of fiber you eat in either quantity or frequency will give your tummy a chance to adjust to the new demands. I'm sure your mate and coworkers will be appreciative as well.

Align Yourself With Other Vegans. You may be the only vegan in your entire family or social circle - can you handle that? You may also feel confused and alone as you make this journey, sometimes enduring ridicule or censure from relatives and friends who don't "get" why you feel compelled to change your diet. Having the support and encouragement of other vegans can be crucial to your success, especially when you are feeling disheartened or fighting cravings. Other vegans have either been where you are and can share their wisdom and experience, or they're right there with you. Either way, by having other vegans around, you won't feel so alone on your journey. There are vegan Meet-Up groups all over the country - many get together and go out for dinner together, or set up pot-lucks. There are also hundreds of online forums and Facebook groups filled with people passionate about the vegan lifestyle.

Eat a Variety of Foods. Unfortunately, lots of people get stuck in food ruts, and eat only what they "like" and are familiar with – over and over and over again. Broaden your food horizons by trying new fruits and vegetables regularly. By "eating the rainbow" (putting mixed colors of food on your plate at each meal), you'll have more fiber, calcium, Vitamin D, Vitamin C, Vitamin B-12, potassium, magnesium, iron, and protein free of saturated fat. Lots of variety means you won't ever get bored with your meals.

Cooking at home is the best way to expose yourself to the vast number of choices available for tasty, nutritious plant based vegan meals.

About These Recipes

The pages of *Why Vegan is the New Black* are filled with great tasting menu ideas created from (mostly) familiar ingredients. Each recipe was selected to provide you with delicious, easy to prepare, and inexpensive things to eat as you begin your transition to a more plant-centered diet. The dishes are not fancy – just good, solid, home style cooking that makes it a lot easier to improve your eating habits.

A few notes on ingredients: All recipes that originally called for chicken or beef broth were revised to use vegan chicken style seasoning powder, "not-chicken" or "not beef" bouillon cubes, or vegetable broth/bouillon cubes. When a recipe sets out a measurement, it is the dry or raw quantity, so you know exactly how much to start with.

Salt used may be kosher or sea salt, with my personal preference being Himalayan pink salt. You may also see references to smoked salt and black salt (kala namak), a salt which adds a slight sulfur smell and an "eggy" flavor to foods cooked with it.

Many of these recipes have been passed from generation to generation in my own family, or were given to me ages ago by friends. Each recipe has been modified to make it meat and dairy free, and every effort has been made to retain the spirit and flavor of the original dish.

Sauces, Marinades and Dressings

Smoky Texas Barbecue Sauce

Makes 4 Cups

Folks in Kansas City, Memphis and Mississippi try to claim the crown for the best barbecue sauce around, but my money is on Texas. While there in the 1980s, I spent months trying this and that, developing what I think is some of the best 'cue sauce ever. Slather this stuff on veggie burgers, vegan ribz, or use it in place of ketchup on fries.

Ingredients

1 cup water
2 cups ketchup
½ cup apple cider vinegar
¾ cup dark brown sugar (packed lightly)
½ cup finely chopped onion
½ cup finely chopped green bell pepper
½ cup finely chopped celery
½ cup finely chopped parsley
2 cloves garlic
1 fresh organic lemon
¼ teaspoon hot pepper sauce
1½ Tablespoons vegan Worcestershire sauce
1½ Tablespoons liquid smoke seasoning
1 teaspoon sea salt
½ teaspoon each dry basil leaves, oregano leaves, and ground cinnamon
2 Tablespoons vegan butter

Instructions

- Put onion, green pepper, celery, parsley and garlic in food processor; blend until smooth.
- Dump mixture into a three quart saucepan. Add ketchup, vinegar, brown sugar and water.
- Ream juice from the lemon, discarding the seeds. Cut off the tips of the lemon and throw the rind and the lemon juice in the pot.
- Add the remaining ingredients, crumbling the oregano and basil leaves between your fingers as you add them to the pot.
- Cook sauce, uncovered, over medium-low heat until reduced to one quart (about 45 minutes). Stir often to prevent sticking.
- Remove from heat and let cool. Store in refrigerator in mason jars, or some other air-tight container for up to seven days.

Fire Tartar Sauce
Serves 4-6

While I was making this the first time, I happened to be playing The Ohio Players 70s CD "FIRE", and it thoroughly inspired me. Everything that came out of the kitchen that day was spicy. This sauce is straight fire, but so good.

Ingredients

½ cup vegan mayonnaise

1 shallot, minced

3 gherkin pickles, minced

¼ teaspoon fresh ground black pepper

1 or more Tablespoons Sriracha sauce

1 teaspoon fresh lemon juice

Instructions

- Combine all ingredients in a small bowl.
- Cover and chill for at least an hour before serving.
- Stores well in refrigerator for up to one week.

Mexican Style Cashew Cheeze Sauce

Makes About 20 Ounces

Use this sauce on vegan quesadillas, nachos, or as a chip dip. It's also great in macaroni and cheese, or grilled cheese sandwiches. Watch how much water you add... start with just a half cup. You may not need much if your cashews are well soaked.

Ingredients

2 cups raw cashews (soaked about 5 hours)

½ cup or more of water

¾ cup nutritional yeast flakes

½ teaspoon ancho chile powder

¼ teaspoon onion powder

¾ teaspoon white pepper

1 teaspoon kosher salt

Instructions

• Drain and rinse cashews.

• Put all ingredients in a high speed blender or food processor, and process until smooth and creamy.

• Taste, and add a bit of cayenne or garlic powder if desired.

Chinese Style Tofu Marinade
Makes One Cup

Makes enough marinade for one 16 oz package of tofu. Dry-fry means with little to no oil in a non-stick skillet to develop a crusty coating on the tofu. Use marinated tofu for snacks, or to top stir-fried vegetables or brown rice.

Ingredients

½ cup low sodium tamari sauce

¼ cup rice wine

1 large clove garlic, minced

½ Tablespoon grated fresh ginger

1 Tablespoon agave nectar

1 16 oz package tofu, pressed to remove extra water

Instructions

• Combine all ingredients except tofu in a small bowl.

• Slice pressed tofu into rectangles or triangles about ¼" thick.

• Heat non-stick skillet over medium. When hot add slices of tofu without crowding the pan.

• Cook until golden brown, then flip and brown the other side.

• Remove from pan and top with marinade.

• Use in place of seitan, tempeh, or meat over rice, or in vegetable stir-fries.

Tahini Salad Dressing
Makes 1.5 Cups

I admit to being a hit or miss salad eater, but a good dressing is always strong motivation.

Ingredients

½ cup sesame tahini

½ cup fresh lemon juice

1 clove garlic (or ½ teaspoon garlic powder)

½ teaspoon sea salt

¼ cup or more of water

Instructions

• Combine all ingredients in blender.

• Blend until smooth and creamy, adding water to reach consistency desired.

• Dressing will thicken when chilled.

• Stores well in refrigerator for up to 10 days.

Ginger & Almond Dressing
Makes 10 Ounces

Sweetness with a little bit of crunch from the almonds.

Ingredients

¼ cup raw almonds

¼ cup almond milk

½ cup water

2 Tablespoons sesame tahini

3 Medjool dates, pitted

1 clove garlic

½" piece of fresh ginger, peeled

Instructions

• Combine all ingredients in blender.

• Blend until smooth.

Easy Everyday Tofu Marinade
Makes 6 Ounces

Makes enough to season one 16 oz package of tofu after pan frying or baking.

Ingredients

½ cup Bragg's liquid aminos

¼ teaspoon rice vinegar

½ large sweet yellow or red onion, minced

5 cloves garlic, crushed

¼ cup water

1 16 oz package tofu, pressed to remove extra water

Instructions

- Combine all ingredients except tofu in blender; blend until smooth.
- Slice pressed tofu into rectangles or triangles about ¼" thick.
- Heat non-stick skillet over medium. When hot, add slices of tofu without crowding the pan.
- Cook until golden brown, then flip and brown the other side.
- Remove from pan and top with marinade. Allow tofu to marinate for about 5 minutes.
- Use in place of seitan, tempeh or meat over rice or in vegetable stir-fries.

Making Vegan Mayonnaise
Makes 20 Servings

Creamy, smooth, with just the right blend of sweet and tart. It's hard to believe there are no eggs in this vegan mayo. Even though it's animal free, mayonnaise is still high in fat, so I wouldn't go crazy with this if your goal is weight loss. Make mayo a few hours before you need to use it so flavors have time to blend.

Ingredients

½ cup sweetened vanilla or plain almond milk

1½ Tablespoons golden flax seeds (ground)

1-2 teaspoons agave nectar

1 teaspoon dry mustard powder

1 teaspoon granulated onion

¼ teaspoon Himalayan pink salt

¼ teaspoon white pepper

1 Tablespoon white wine vinegar

1 Tablespoon fresh lemon juice

¾ to 1 cup expeller pressed grape seed oil

Instructions

- Add almond milk and flax seed meal to blender. Blend at med-high speed for 60-90 seconds, or until all the little bits of flax meal are gone.
- Add the lemon juice and vinegar. Blend for 15 seconds. Then add the granulated onion, mustard powder, white pepper, agave nectar, and pink salt. Blend for another 30 seconds.
- Reduce blender speed and leave running. Remove top at center and start slowly pouring in the grape seed oil. At a certain point you'll see the mayo start thickening. Add a bit more oil and continue blending until mixture reaches thickness you desire.
- Spoon into clean glass jar with airtight top, and refrigerate immediately.

Mississippi Secret Sauce
Makes About 1 Cup

My maternal grandmother was born and raised in Egypt, Mississippi. We always got a kick out of telling people "my grandmother is Egyptian!" She shared many recipes with me over the years (some of which appear in this book), as I would spend almost every waking moment with her during summer vacations. She taught me to crochet, as well as how to make this "Secret Sauce" that she'd keep in the refrigerator and bring to family barbecues in recycled ketchup bottles. This sauce goes well on any type of vegan sandwich, burger, vegetables, or meats for the non-vegans in your family. It also goes great on tacos or burritos in place of salsa, as salad dressing, or in place of tartar sauce on your tempeh fish. Refrigerate for up to three weeks, if it lasts that long.

Ingredients

¼ cup bottled chili sauce

¼ cup of thick ketchup

1 Tablespoon of vegan Worcestershire sauce

1 teaspoon spicy brown or Creole mustard

1 cup vegan mayonnaise

1 teaspoon fresh ground black pepper

½ teaspoon Cajun seasoning

½ teaspoon hot pepper sauce (I like Sriracha, Grandmom used Tabasco)

1 teaspoon onion powder

½ teaspoon garlic powder

2 teaspoons light brown sugar

3 Tablespoons fresh lemon juice

Instructions

- Dump all the ingredients in a blender and let it whir until everything is evenly mixed.
- Taste sauce, and make seasoning adjustments as required.
- Store in the refrigerator.

Aunt Helen's Tartar Sauce
Makes About 1 Cup

Watching my aunt whip this up, I discovered that making tartar sauce is super easy, and the fresh taste is far better than any commercial product I've ever tasted. Use it with your tempeh or tofu fish, as a mix-in for potato salad, or even as a sandwich spread.

Ingredients

¾ cup vegan mayonnaise

1 teaspoon Dijon mustard

¼ teaspoon cayenne pepper

3 Tablespoons finely chopped green onions (white and pale green parts only)

3 Tablespoons minced fresh parsley

1 Tablespoon sweet pickle relish

Instructions

• Whisk mayo, mustard and cayenne together until well blended.
• Stir in the green onions, parsley and pickle relish.
• Allow to sit in refrigerator for an hour or more before use.
• Store in airtight container and use it within a week.

Vegan Buttermilk Ranch Dressing
Makes 2 Cups

I have to admit I am not a big salad eater. Something about all that chopping, washing, rinsing, slicing and dicing only to end up with a plate of rabbit food does not really appeal to me. However, if someone else makes it, or I dump it out of a bag, I'll eat a huge serving. Weird, I know. Salad, no matter how it gets in front of me, is always better with the rich, creamy flavor of ranch dressing. This recipe works great as a dip for Buffalo Wangz. Add a few extra tablespoons of sour cream and it makes a great dip for raw crudities. Cover it up tight and it will keep well for at least 4-5 days.

Ingredients

½ cup unsweetened almond milk

1½ teaspoons fresh lemon juice

½ cup vegan sour cream

1 cup vegan mayonnaise

¼ cup olive oil

¼ cup apple cider vinegar

1 clove garlic, chopped

1 teaspoon dry mustard

1 teaspoon dried dill

1 teaspoon dried thyme

½ teaspoon sea salt

½ teaspoon fresh ground black pepper

Dash of Tabasco or other hot sauce

¼ cup chopped parsley

Instructions

• Add lemon juice to nut milk and stir. Let sit on counter for 5-10 minutes to curdle before use (this is your "buttermilk").

• Put sour cream, buttermilk, mayonnaise, olive oil, vinegar, garlic, dry mustard, dill, thyme, salt, pepper and pepper sauce into blender, and process until smooth.

• Remove to serving container and stir in the chopped parsley.

Agave Dill Vinaigrette

Makes About 2 Cups

Whip this dressing up in the blender in seconds. Its flavors are very complimentary to salads that have nuts, seeds, or fruit in addition to raw vegetables. Dressing keeps in the fridge for about a week if stored in an airtight container.

Ingredients

½ cup balsamic vinegar

¼ cup agave or maple syrup

4 cloves garlic, chopped

1 Tablespoon dried dill

1 cup extra virgin olive oil

Kosher salt

Fresh ground black pepper

Instructions

- Put the vinegar, agave, garlic and dill into the blender, and blend until smooth. With blender still running, add the olive oil in a thin stream until dressing is emulsified.
- Season to taste with salt and fresh ground pepper.

Breakfast Ideas

Biscuits and Sausage Gravy
Serves 4

A Southern favorite, redone vegan without the saturated fat and cholesterol. Start with the Fluffy Whole Wheat Buttermilk Biscuits recipe, then top them with this gravy. Yum!

Ingredients

½ cup all purpose unbleached flour

1½ cups water

3 cups soy or almond milk

4 vegan sausage substitute patties

½ not-beef bouillon cube

½ cup vegetable oil

1 teaspoon seasoned salt

1 teaspoon fresh ground black pepper

Chopped green onions (optional)

Instructions

- Sauté your favorite vegan sausage until fully cooked and lightly browned. Crumble into sausage into smaller pieces, and set aside.
- Add oil to large skillet and stir in flour and black pepper over low heat. Continuously stir to prevent burning, until the mixture is brown and creamy.
- Slowly pour in the soy milk while stirring. Continue to stir until gravy is creamy and flour/milk are blended.
- Add in the crumbled vegan sausage and let simmer 3-5 minutes, adding more warm water as needed to maintain consistency.
- Serve hot over baking powder or whole wheat biscuits.

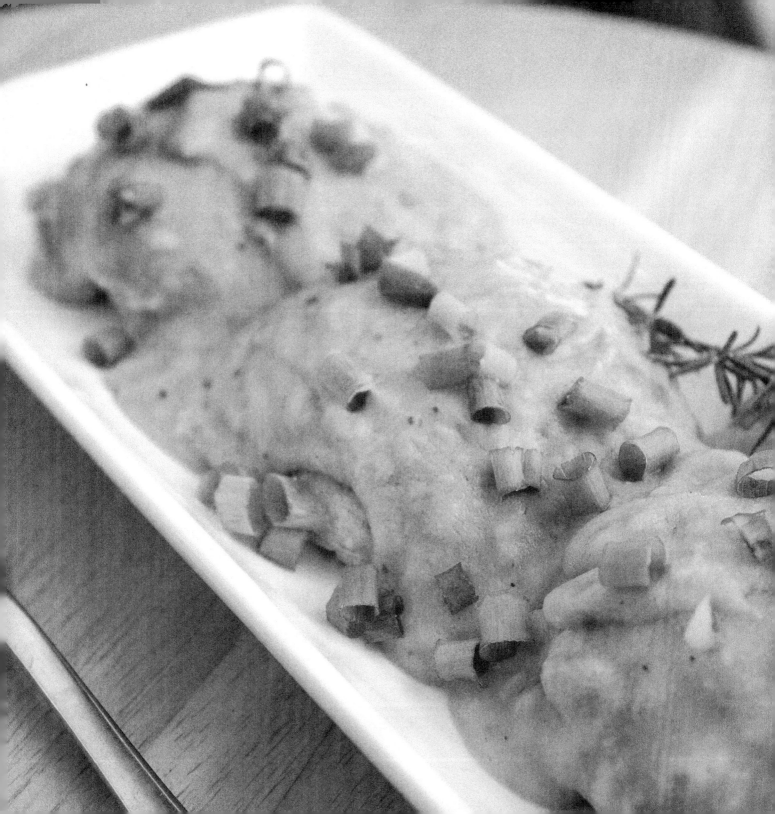

Egg Free Omelet
Makes 4 Servings

Vegans can still enjoy omelets stuffed with vegetables, cheese (vegan), and even vegan meats if you like. This quick to prepare recipe will serve four. Add a serving of fruit, grits, or maybe hash browns, and you have a meal fit for a king!

Ingredients

1 shallot
1 carton Extra Firm silken tofu (non-GMO and organic)
2 rounded Tablespoons nutritional yeast
½ teaspoon tofu seasoning blend
¼ teaspoon The Vegg® powder
1½ teaspoons black salt (kala namak)
2 Tablespoons olive oil
½ cup unsweetened almond milk
½ cup chickpea flour
1½ Tablespoons arrowroot powder (can substitute corn or potato starch)

For Omelet Stuffing

1 Tablespoon vegan butter or olive oil
4 cups baby spinach leaves
4 green onions, chopped small
1 Fresno pepper, seeded and minced
8 mushrooms, sliced thin
½ yellow or red bell pepper, minced
½ red onion, minced

Instructions

- Place tofu in blender, add shallot, nutritional yeast, olive oil, turmeric, almond milk, The Vegg®, tofu seasoning blend, and 1 teaspoon kala namak. Puree until smooth.
- Add the chickpea flour and arrowroot, and mix again for about 20 seconds, scraping sides as you go to make sure everything is well mixed.
- Batter should be thick and pasty, but spreadable. It does not pour, you have to scoop it with a spoon. If the mixture is TOO thick, thin it slightly with 1-2 Tablespoons of water.
- Set batter aside and prep your filling mix.
- Put 1-2 teaspoons olive oil in 10" non-stick skillet. When hot, add the onion, mushrooms, and peppers and sauté until soft. Add spinach and green onions, stirring until spinach is wilted. Remove from pan to a bowl.

- Return same pan to stove over medium heat, Spray with cooking spray if needed. When pan is hot again, add about ¼ of the batter to pan and spread it quickly and evenly with back of spoon. Your goal is to make a 7-8" circle.
- Let batter cook over medium heat 4-5 minutes. Shake pan to loosen omelet, then carefully turn it over to cook the other side.
- When second side has cooked about 30 seconds, add your vegan cheese of choice and stuffing to one half of the omelet.
- Sprinkle with portion of remaining black salt. Flip other side of omelet over so that it tops the stuffing and cheese. Gently shake pan to loosen omelet, then side it out onto a plate to serve.
- Top with avocado, salsa, or additional vegan cheese.

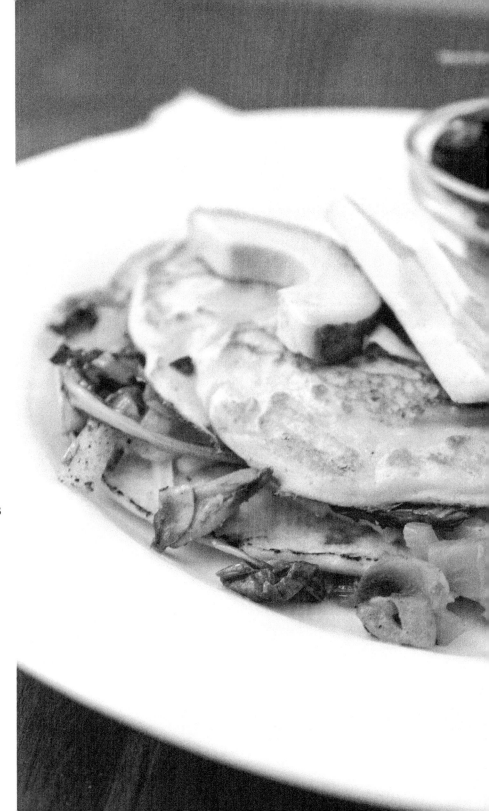

Southern Style Baking Powder Biscuits
Makes 1 Dozen

One of the things I remember my grandmother stressing when she taught me how to make biscuits was to handle the dough as delicately as possible. Her touch was so light, and her biscuits were fluffy and melt-in-your-mouth delicious every time. Though I eventually got the hang of it, my first tries produced something more like a hockey puck than anything edible.

Ingredients

2 cups all purpose unbleached flour

3 teaspoons baking powder

½ teaspoon Himalayan pink salt

4 Tablespoons cold vegan butter-style spread

¾ to 1 cup cold plant milk

Instructions

- Preheat oven to 450 degrees.
- Grease a baking sheet.
- Sift dry ingredients together into large bowl.
- Cut butter into chunks, then mix with pastry blender until fine mealy texture forms.
- Stir milk into dry mixture, adding a few sprinkles more if needed to make a soft dough.
- Toss lightly on a floured board or counter until surface of dough is smooth and covered with flour.
- Gently roll or press out ½" thick, and cut with floured biscuit cutter.
- Bake for 13-14 minutes.
- Brush with melted butter spread while hot.

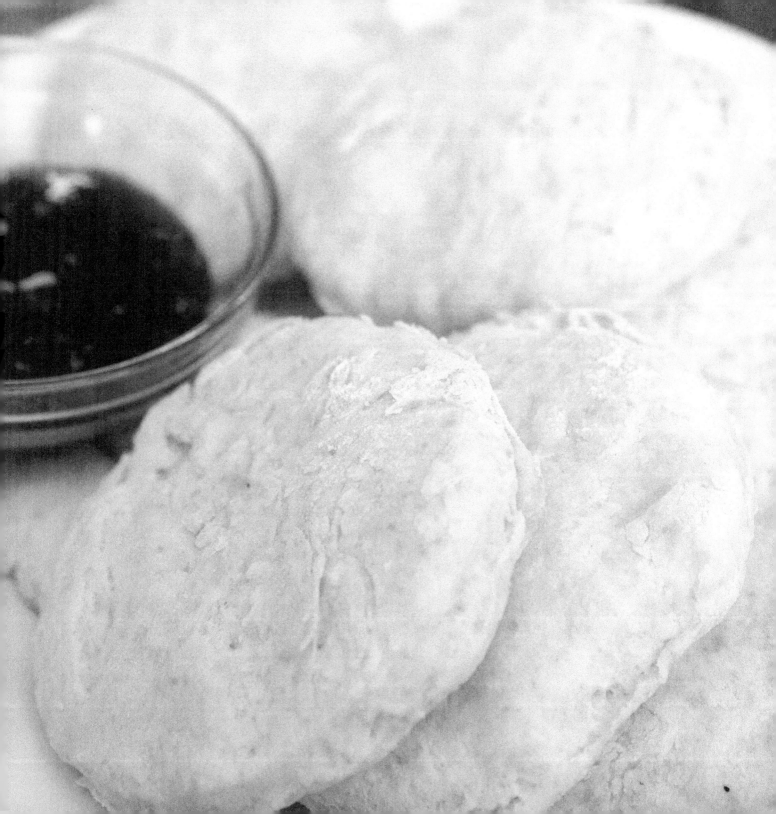

Tofu Scramble Seasoning Mix
Makes 5 Ounces

Achieving the perfect balance of seasoning for tofu scrambles is a tricky business. After trying many experiments, a wide variety of seasonings (achieving a wide variety of results), I found that starting with a simple base is the best approach. Prepare this blend and keep it in a recycled jar, ready for use. Add any vegetables you have handy in the fridge if you want.

Ingredients

½ cup nutritional yeast flakes

2 teaspoons black salt (kala namak)

2 teaspoons onion powder

1 teaspoons garlic powder

1 teaspoon white pepper

1 teaspoon turmeric

½ teaspoon cayenne pepper

Instructions

• Put all ingredients in a food processor or blender, and whir until a fine powder is formed.

• Store in airtight container for up to six months.

To Use Seasoning Blend

Melt 2 Tablespoons vegan butter in large non-stick skillet over medium heat. Add onions, shallots or vegetables. Once vegetables are tender, add crumbled tofu and 2 rounded Tablespoons of seasoning mixture.
Scramble tofu around gently with spatula as you would eggs. Let it sit in pan for 5-7 minutes, then scramble again. Taste and add black pepper, additional salt, cheese or more cayenne. Serve hot.

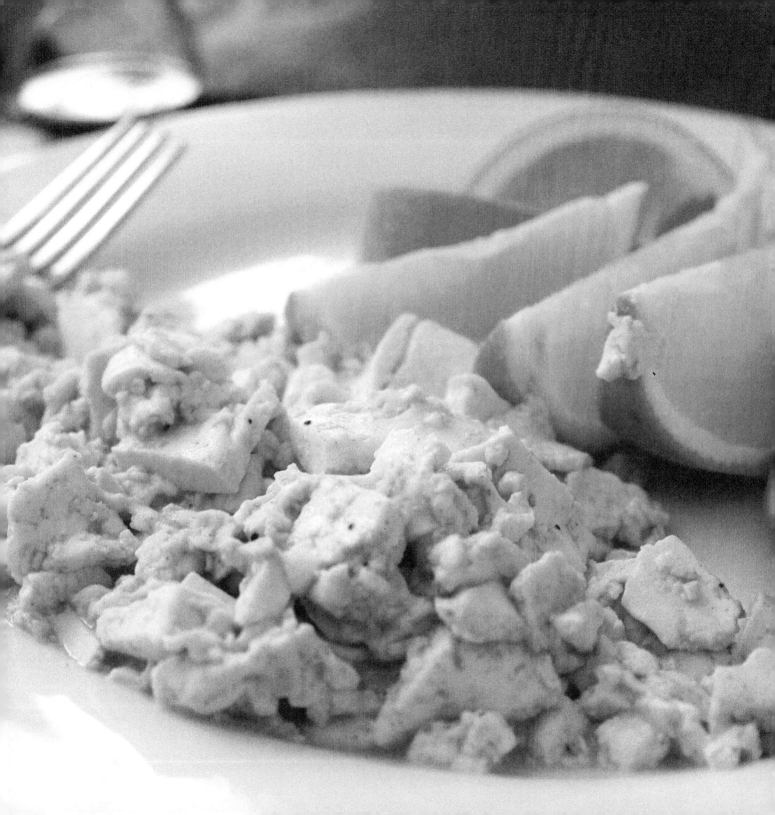

Spicy Scramble With Mushrooms, Kale and Tomatoes
Serves 2-3

This gourmet scramble is perfect for company because it looks fancy and tastes great. Any hot pepper will do here, but I prefer red Fresno peppers or ripe jalapeños (which are also red). Fresno peppers are very similar to jalapeños in shape and in size, but they can be even hotter. Mild-tasting Lacinto kale and cherry tomatoes boost the nutritional profile of this hearty breakfast, while adding great color and flavor.

Ingredients

2 Tablespoons vegan butter or olive oil

1 shallot, diced

1 clove garlic, diced

1 green onion, chopped

1-2 Fresno peppers, seeded and diced

4-6 cremini mushrooms, washed and sliced

1 14 oz package water packed medium to medium-firm tofu, pressed lightly

1 cup minced lacinto kale leaves (about 5 leaves, stems removed)

⅓ cup nutritional yeast flakes

2-3 Tablespoons Bragg's liquid aminos

8 organic grape tomatoes, sliced in quarters lengthwise

¼ cup vegan mozzarella or cheddar shreds

Fresh ground black pepper

Instructions

• Over medium heat, add oil to large non-stick skillet. When hot, add shallot, mushrooms, green onion, diced pepper, and garlic to the pan. Let cook about 1 minute.

• Crumble tofu into pan. Add ⅓ of the nutritional yeast, 1 Tablespoon of Bragg's, and a few shakes of black pepper. Reduce heat to low and allow mixture to cook about 3 minutes.

• Using spatula, lift mixture from the bottom of pan and gently incorporate seasonings into tofu. Let cook undisturbed another 2-3 minutes.

• Mix in minced kale, then add another ⅓ of the nutritional yeast, 2 teaspoons of Bragg's aminos, and a few more shakes of black pepper. Allow mixture to cook for another 3-4 minutes. A crust will form on the bottom of the pan, that's fine.

• Toss in your quartered grape tomatoes, the rest of the nutritional years, aminos and another few shakes of black pepper. Toss in the cheese and mix thoroughly with spatula, again lifting from the bottom.

• Serve hot.

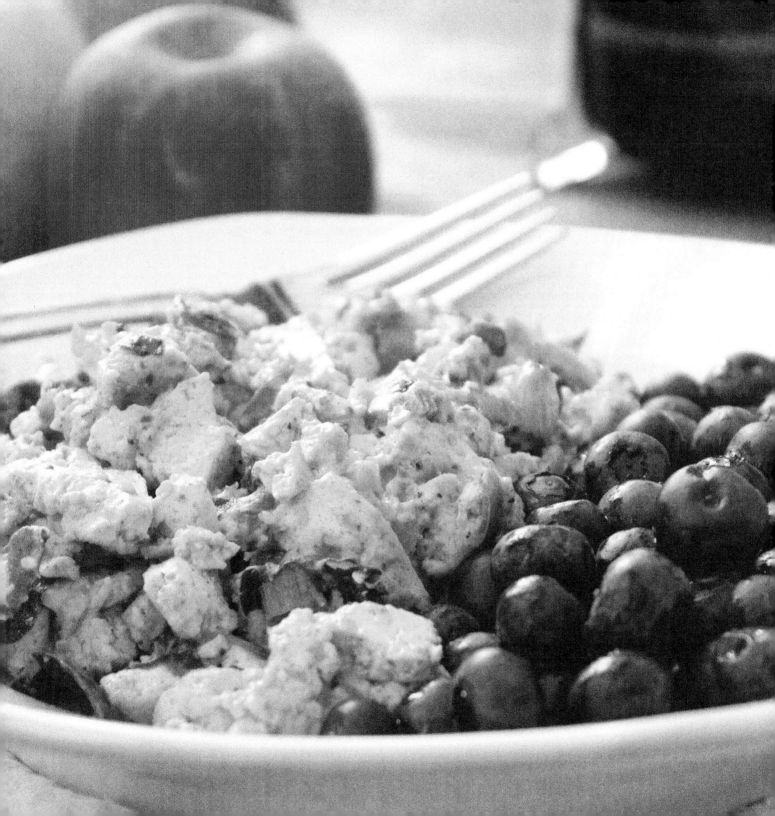

Fluffy Whole Wheat Biscuits
Makes 10-12

Perfect with tofu scramble for breakfast, for sliders as lunch, as a side with dinner, or warm with jam and coffee as a snack. To me any time of the day or night is the right time for biscuits. The number of biscuits you end up with will vary, depending upon the size of your cutter. I use a small glass and make mine about 2½-3 inches in diameter.

Ingredients

1½ cups unbleached flour

1½ cups whole wheat flour

1½ Tablespoons aluminum free baking powder

½ teaspoon baking soda

1 teaspoon sea salt

6 Tablespoons vegan buttery spread, chilled and cut into chunks

10 oz chilled soy or almond milk

‡ Chill buttery spread and plant milk for a few minutes in the freezer for best results.

Instructions

- Preheat oven to 425. Spray baking sheet with non-stick spray.
- Combine flours, salt, baking soda, and baking powder in large mixing bowl.
- Add chilled vegan butter, and cut in with a pastry blender until fine crumbly texture.
- Pour in cold soy or almond milk a little at a time, mixing until all flour is incorporated, but dough is easy to handle. Do not over-wet.
- Remove from bowl onto a lightly floured board or counter. Knead with fingertips lightly 6-8 times, then press dough into a ¾-1" high square.
- Cut biscuits and place on prepared baking sheet, leaving at least ½" space between them. Brush tops with melted vegan butter.
- Bake until golden brown, about 10-12 minutes. Cooled leftovers can be stored in an airtight container in the refrigerator.

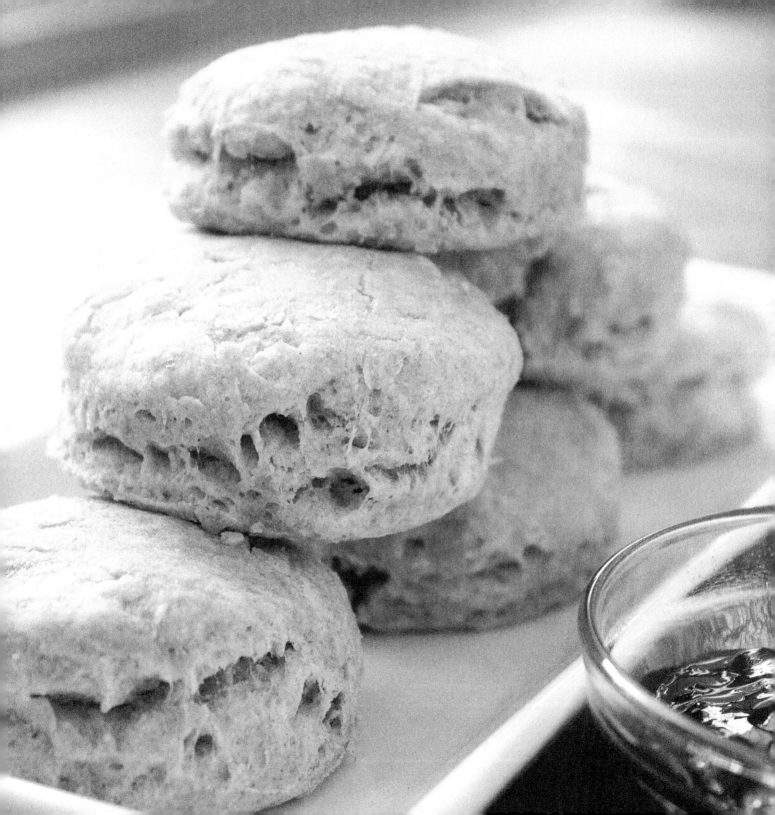

Refrigerator Oats with Chia Seeds
Serves 4

Chia seeds boast Omega-3 fatty acids (good for your heart and joints), protein, antioxidants, magnesium, and potassium - plus, they're high in fiber. Top it off with chopped walnuts and blueberries for a powerful dose of goodness to get your day started off right.

Ingredients

1½ cups steel-cut organic oats

1½ cups plant milk of your choice

3 Tablespoons chia seeds

¼ teaspoon ground cardamom

½ teaspoon vanilla extract

¼ teaspoon ground ginger

½ teaspoon ground cinnamon

¼ teaspoon ground nutmeg

3 Medjool dates, pitted and chopped

1 cup fresh blueberries

4 Tablespoons chopped walnuts

Instructions

- Combine oats, plant milk, chia seeds, cardamom, vanilla, ginger, cinnamon, nutmeg and chopped walnuts in large wide-mouth Mason jar.
- Stir well, close lid, and place in refrigerator before bed (overnight).
- In the morning, stir contents of jar and divide into four bowls. Sprinkle each serving with ¼ cup of blueberries and 2 teaspoons of chopped nuts.

Make Your Own Granola
Makes 4-5 Cups

This is not a low calorie breakfast, but it tastes really good and travels well. It's great for eating with fruit and nut milk for breakfast, but also mixes well into coconut or soy yogurt for snack time. One serving is about a quarter cup, but I always measure out double that for myself.

Ingredients

4 cups quick-cooking oats

½ cup chopped nuts (walnuts, almonds, cashews or a combination thereof)

¼ cup dark molasses

¼ cup agave nectar

1½ teaspoons ground cinnamon

2 teaspoons vanilla extract

Non-stick butter flavored cooking spray

Instructions

- Preheat oven to 300 degrees. Coat two baking pans (the type with edges) with cooking spray.
- Mix all ingredients together in large bowl. Spread mixture about ½" thick in both pans
- Bake 35-40 minutes, opening oven to shake pans every 10 minutes or so to make sure granola browns evenly.
- Cool, then remove from trays and place in airtight containers.
- For freshest taste and best crunch, use within two weeks.

Oatmeal Walnut Pancakes
Serves 8

Children love these pancakes, and you'll love the fiber, protein and good Omega-3 fats they'll get. Easy to whip up, you can get a nutritious hot breakfast on the table in less than 30 minutes.

Ingredients

3 cups old-fashioned or rolled oats

⅔ cup chopped walnuts

3 Tablespoons agave nectar

1 teaspoon egg replacer powder

1 teaspoon vanilla extract

¼ teaspoon ground cinnamon

½ teaspoon salt

3½ cups water

Instructions

- Put everything into a food processor or high speed blender, and blend until smooth.
- Heat large non-stick skillet over medium about two minutes, or until ⅛th teaspoon of water stays in a ball and rolls around your pan.
- Pour about ¼ cup of batter into the pan for each pancake. Once bubbles form and pop in the middle, flip pancake over and cook another minute or two.
- Remove to warmed plate (250 degree oven) until you have made all your pancakes.
- Serve warm with favorite toppings such as sliced banana, berries, maple syrup, or vegan butter. Whipped coconut cream topping (page 171) makes breakfast extraordinary.

Blueberry Pancakes
Serves 3-4

If blueberries are out of season, frozen organic berries work very well, too. Just defrost them in a strainer so that extra water drains away before use.

Ingredients

1½ cups whole wheat flour

½ teaspoon sea salt

2 teaspoons aluminum free baking powder

1 cup fresh or frozen blueberries

1½ cups plant milk

1 Tablespoon coconut oil

2 teaspoons apple cider vinegar

2 Tablespoons agave nectar

½ teaspoon vanilla extract

Non-stick butter flavored cooking spray or vegan butter for pan

Instructions

- Combine the flour, salt and baking powder in a large bowl.
- In another smaller bowl, combine the plant milk, vinegar, vanilla and agave. Pour into dry ingredients and mix well. The batter will be rather thick.
- Gently mix in blueberries by hand to prevent them from bursting.
- Apply a thin coating of the vegan butter or buttery spray to skillet. Heat heavy skillet over medium heat.
- Pour about one-third cup of the batter into pan for each pancake. Cook until golden brown then flip and cook second side (about 3½-4 minutes per side).
- Serve with pure maple syrup.

Breakfast Soft Tacos
Serves 2

A great way to use leftover baked or boiled potatoes, as well as leftover tofu scramble. Wrap your tacos up in foil for a great "to-go" breakfast you can eat in the car.

Ingredients

4 Artisan corn tortillas

1 Tablespoon olive oil

2 large potatoes (boiled or previously baked)

Tofu scramble (½ recipe)

2 Tablespoons pico de gallo or salsa

2 Tablespoons diced green chilies

½ cup vegan cheddar cheeze strips

Instructions

- Wrap tortillas in foil and warm in oven at 325 degrees for 8-10 minutes.
- Dice potatoes and brown in non-stick skillet with oil. When toasty brown on all sides, stir in pico de gallo and tofu scramble. Mix well and heat for 2-3 minutes until hot.
- Place two tortillas on each plate and fill each with ¼ of the filling mixture.
- Top with cheeze and additional salsa, if desired.

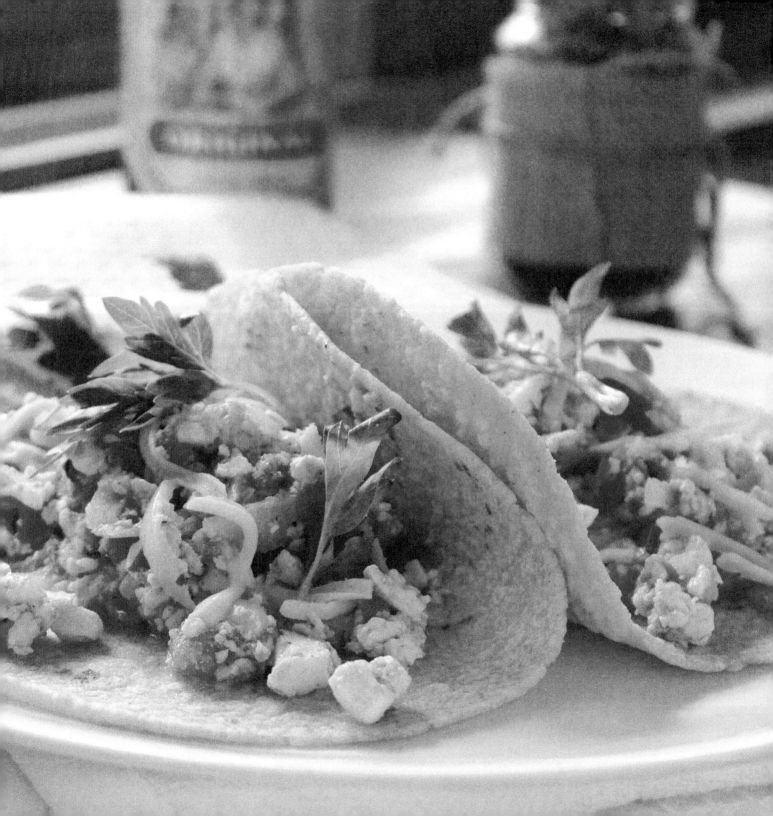

Peachy Keen Breakfast Smoothie
Serves 2

High in vitamin A, vitamin C, potassium, and vitamin B-6, you can enjoy this deliciously satisfying smoothie without worrying much about calories. The Peachy Keen comes in right around 300 per serving.

Ingredients

2½ cups of peach chunks (peeled)

1 cup baby carrots

½ cup plain almond or soy yogurt

1 frozen banana

¼ cup old-fashioned rolled oats

1 cup coconut water

2 teaspoons agave nectar

3-5 ice cubes

Instructions

• Put everything into a high speed blender, and blend until smooth (about 30-45 seconds).

Sunrise Green Smoothie
Serves 1-2

Many people struggle to meet the suggested daily minimum of four to six servings of green leafy vegetables, and three to four servings of fresh fruit. Solving such a dilemma can be easy with a nutritious fruit and vegetable based green smoothie.

Ingredients

1 cup tightly packed curly kale or spinach, washed

2 Tablespoons fresh parsley leaves

½ a green apple, chopped

1 small ripe banana, peeled and cut into chunks

¼ ripe avocado, peeled and chopped (½ cup)

½ cup cucumber (peeled and chopped)

1 celery stalk, chopped

1 cup cold coconut water

4-5 ice cubes

Instructions

• Place the kale/spinach, parsley, apple, banana, avocado, and cucumber or celery in blender.

• Add the coconut water and 4-5 ice cubes. Blend on high speed for 60 seconds until thick, smooth and green.

• Try adding one or two of the following for variety: romaine lettuce, fresh orange or tangerine slices, green melon chunks, kefir, peeled kiwi fruit, almonds, goji berry powder, fresh basil leaves, zucchini, fresh mint leaves, acai berries, chia or flax seeds (soaked), coconut oil, a few blueberries, spirulina, pea protein powder, chlorella, peanut or almond butter or powder, fresh grated ginger.

Banana Berry Chocolate Blast
Serves 1-2

1 cup nut or grain milk
2 frozen bananas, cut into chunks
½ cup pineapple chunks (fresh or canned in juice)
5-6 frozen strawberries
2 Tablespoons unsweetened cocoa powder
1 Tablespoon agave nectar

Pour milk into the blender first. Add cocoa and then fruit. Put cover on and blend until smooth.

Yogurt Cinnaberry Smoothie
Serves 1-2

6-8 oz carton blueberry, vanilla or plain soy, coconut or almond yogurt
6 oz nut or grain milk
1 Tablespoon agave nectar
½ to 1 teaspoon ground Ceylon cinnamon
2 cups frozen organic blueberries

Combine the yogurt, milk, agave and cinnamon in a blender until mixed thoroughly. Add the blueberries and blend until smooth.

‡ Ceylon cinnamon is reported to be helpful in stabilizing blood sugar in diabetics and pre-diabetics in doses of up to 1½ teaspoons per day, for up to six weeks a pop. The added nutritional boost of blueberries makes this a high value energy booster.

Date Carob & Banana Smoothie
Serves 1-2

3-4 Medjool dates, pitted and soaked
1 cup nut or grain milk
1 frozen banana, cut in chunks
3-4 Tablespoons carob or cocoa powder
1 vanilla bean or ½ teaspoon vanilla

Place dates in a small bowl with just enough
water to cover. Let them soak 15-20 minutes,
then drain. In blender, combine the dates,
nut milk, banana, carob or cocoa powder and
vanilla bean. Blend until smooth.

Chocolate PB Banana Smoothie
Serves 2

½ cup nut or grain milk
½ cup silken tofu
⅓ cup peanut butter
2 fresh bananas, frozen and sliced
2 Tablespoons chocolate syrup
6 ice cubes

Combine the rice milk, tofu and peanut butter
in a blender. Add the bananas, chocolate syrup
and ice cubes. Blend until smooth, about 30 to
40 seconds. Makes 2 servings.

Fruity Tofu Smoothie
Serves 1-2

½ cup apple juice
6 oz frozen vanilla soy or almond yogurt
4 ounces (½ cup) soft tofu, drained and pressed
1 cup fresh or frozen strawberries or peaches
1 banana, peeled and broken into chunks
1 teaspoon agave nectar or maple syrup
5 ice cubes
Fresh whole berries for garnish (optional)

Place all ingredients into blender. Blend on high until smooth, about 30-40 seconds.

‡ Good way to boost your protein intake if you struggle with meeting your daily requirement. Using almond yogurt and tofu, this smoothie delivers about 16 grams of protein.

Vital Greens Smoothie
Serves 1-2

1 blender container loosely filled with vital or deep greens mix (spinach, baby kale and chard)
½ large banana
1 Tablespoon raw pumpkin seeds
¾ to 1 cup nut or grain milk
3 oz (about ¼ of a can) frozen pineapple juice concentrate
3 cubes ice

Blend until smooth. Note: apple or orange juice concentrate can be used in place of pineapple juice. Be sure it's unsweetened.

‡ Earthbound Farms brand of vital greens or deep greens is popular on the West Coast, but similar bundles of baby greens are sold nationwide under other brand names.

Sweet Potato Muffins
Makes 1 Dozen

Did you know that the humble little sweet potato was ranked the number one most nutritious of ALL vegetables? Yup. Nutritionists at the Center for Science in the Public Interest gave the sweet potato high points for protein, vitamin A, iron, calcium, dietary fiber and its complex carbohydrate content.

Ingredients

1 large (¾-1 pound) sweet potato
2 Tablespoons vegan butter spread
Pinch of salt
2 vegan eggs, prepared
½ cup almond milk
1 teaspoon baking powder
2 cups unbleached all purpose flour

Instructions

- Peel sweet potato and cut it into chunks. Steam or boil it in as little water as possible until thoroughly cooked and soft throughout.
- Preheat oven to 400 degrees.
- Place sweet potato in food processor or blender, and process until there are no lumpy chunks. Add vegan butter, a pinch of salt, and mix well.
- Add vegan eggs, almond milk, and baking powder; mix thoroughly.
- Start adding flour a bit at a time until a soft batter forms. Do not add so much that your dough becomes stiff.
- Line muffin cups with paper liners, and fill each about ¾ full.
- Bake muffins for 25-30 minutes, or until light golden brown.

Entrées, Light Meals and Sides
For Lunch or Dinner

Mexicali Red Rice
Serves 4

In Texas the blend of Mexican and Texan flavors is called "Tex-Mex", so I think it only fitting that we have "Mexi-Cali", right? I love red rice and can eat this stuff for breakfast, lunch and dinner. If you don't like or can't handle spicy food, leave out the jalapeño and be sure to purchase tomatoes with mild green chilies.

Ingredients

2 cups long grain white rice (I use Jasmine)

2 12 oz cans tomatoes with green chilies, drained of juice

1 white onion, quartered

3 cloves garlic

1 not-chicken bouillon cube

2 cups not-chicken or vegetable broth

½ cup vegetable oil

½ teaspoon sea salt (or to taste)

¼ teaspoon chili powder

½ teaspoon fresh ground black pepper

1½ cups frozen peas and carrots

2 sprigs fresh cilantro

2 Tablespoons olive oil

2 Tablespoons vegan butter

Instructions

• Rinse and drain the rice.

• Dump can of tomatoes, onion, garlic, jalapeño and 2 cups of broth in blender and puree until smooth. Pour into measuring cup, then add broth to total four cups of liquid.

• In large skillet, heat oils and rice. Stirring frequently, sauté rice until it turns golden brown (about 8-10 minutes)

• Slowly pour pureed tomato/broth mixture over rice, add bouillon cube, peas and carrots, salt and pepper. Stir just once or twice.

• Bring mixture to a boil, throw in cilantro sprigs, then cover and simmer over low heat for 15-20 minutes.

• Leave top on another 8-10 minutes before removing to allow rice to finish steaming and become fluffy.

• Remove cilantro sprigs and serve as a side dish, or use it in burritos. Works well for breakfast with tofu scramble.

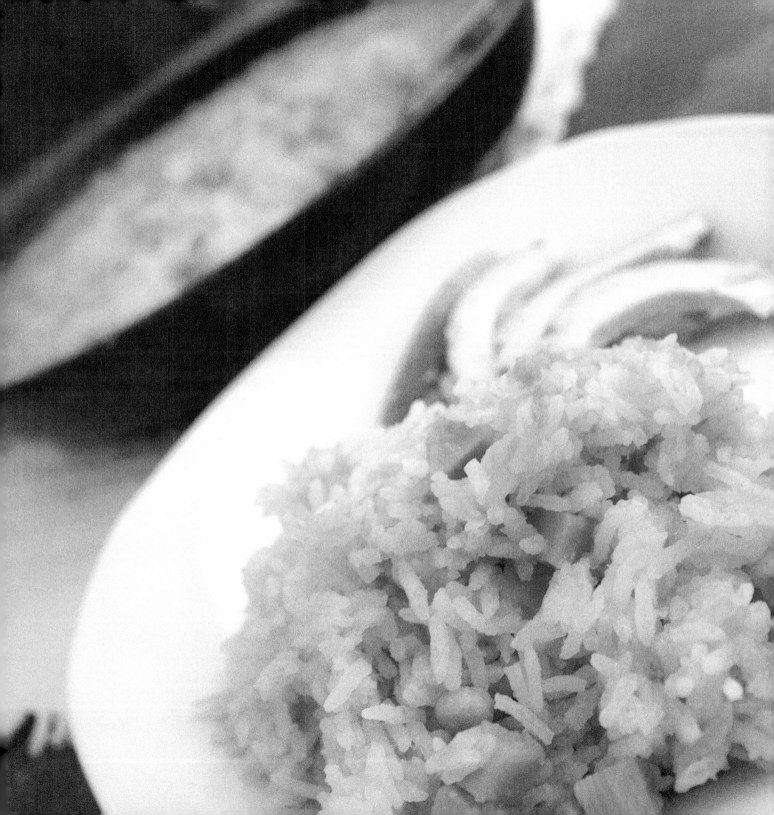

Hearty Vegetable Stock
Makes 4 Quarts

Vegetable stock is a staple item in the vegan or vegetarian kitchen, and serves as the star ingredient in many of the following recipes. Using commercial stock in a pinch is a convenient option. However, the most flavorful results are obtained when you make your own vegetable stock - and you'll also know exactly what's in it.

Ingredients

5 large onions, cut in half

10 organic carrots, scrubbed and cut into thirds

8 organic tomatoes, washed and quartered

1 bunch parsley, rinsed well

1-2 cloves garlic, minced

5 celery stalks, washed and cut into thirds

1 bay leaf

2 sprigs fresh thyme

10 black peppercorns

1 leek, cut and rinsed thoroughly (optional)

16 cups cold water

Instructions

- Combine all ingredients in large stock pot and bring to a boil.
- Reduce heat to low, and simmer for 60-75 minutes.
- Turn off heat and let pot sit with cover on for another 30 minutes. Remove any scum which may form on the top of the pot, then strain into airtight container.
- Use within 3 days or freeze.

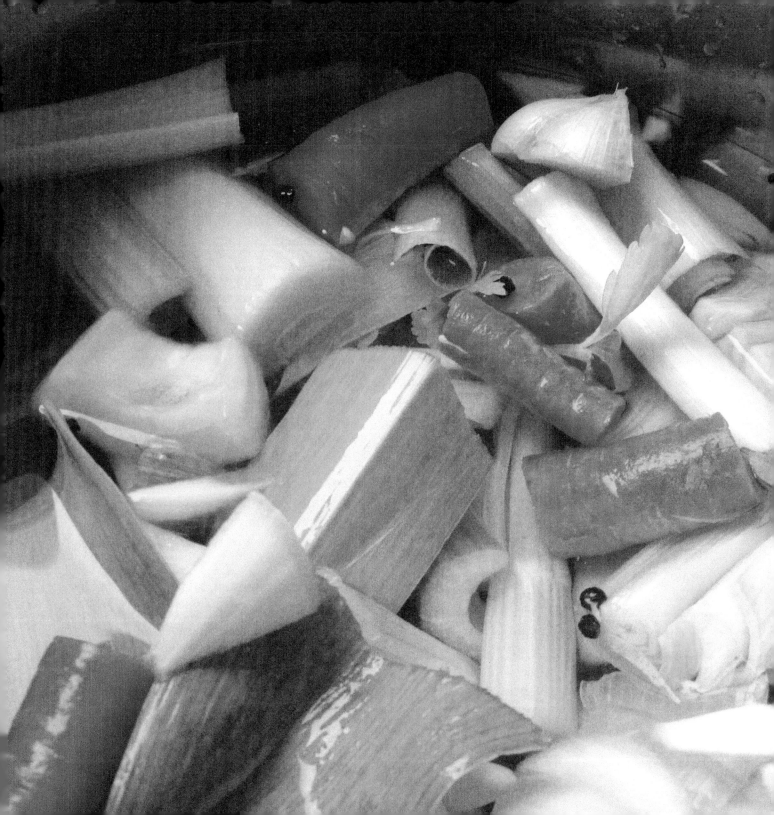

Pancit Bihon with Soy Curls
Serves 8

The noodles used in Filipino dishes are attributed to the early influence of the Chinese – many of the dishes use similar ingredients and as a result, have similar flavors. This is my take on a traditional Filipino dish served at pot lucks, parties and dinners.

Ingredients

1 12-14 oz package of thin rice stick noodles (should say bihon on the package)
½ package soy curls
1 cup water
1 teaspoon vegan chicken style seasoning
1 teaspoon sea salt
3 Tablespoons grape seed or peanut oil
4 cloves garlic, peeled and chopped
1 large yellow onion, sliced thin and cut in half
4 stalks celery, sliced thin on the diagonal
4 carrots, cut into thin strips, then into pieces about ½" long
1 package Sazon Goya con Cilantro y Achiote
1 Tablespoon double black soy sauce
1 cup water
2 Tablespoons vegan fish sauce (sold at Asian markets)
2 cups long beans, cut into ½" pieces
4 cups shredded cabbage
1 red bell pepper, julienned into ½" pieces
1 cup snow peas, trimmed (about 20-25)
4 cups vegetable broth (or equivalent not-chicken seasoning and water)

1 teaspoon fresh ground black pepper (or to taste)
4 green onions, cut in half lengthwise and cut into 1" strips

Instructions

- Measure out approximately half an eight ounce package of soy curls into large bowl. Dissolve chicken-style flavoring in 1 cup warm water, then pour over soy curls. Stir, and let sit 20 minutes to absorb the flavoring.

- Remove bihon noodles from package and place into large bowl. Fill bowl with water and allow noodles to soak and soften for 5 minutes; remove to tray and cover so they stay moist.

- In the meantime wash and chop vegetables and set aside. Combine soy sauce, 1 cup water, Sazon Goya and vegan fish sauce in a small bowl.

- After soy curls have finished soaking, drain in colander, squeezing gently to remove excess liquid. Cut soy curls into 1-2" strips.

- Heat oil in large heavy saucepan or wok, and sauté garlic and onions for about 30 seconds. Add celery and carrots, and cook another minute or two until softened.
- Add the soaked soy curls and mix well. Add the sauce mixture and 3 cups of the vegetable or not-chicken broth, and simmer for about 15 minutes.
- Add shredded cabbage, long beans, and red pepper; mix well. Allow vegetables to cook over low heat for about five minutes, stirring occasionally. Add salt and pepper to taste.
- Drain water from soaked noodles. If you prefer short noodles, you can use kitchen scissors and cut noodles into 2-3" pieces and drop into a bowl.
- Make sure heat is on low. Add noodles to the pan and mix all ingredients together well. Add your remaining cup of broth, cover, and barely simmer for about 5 minutes. Noodles will readily absorb the liquid, but if it starts looking dry, add ¼ cup water.
- Turn off heat, add snow peas and stir. Return top to pan. Let mixture sit and steam for another five minutes before serving.
- Garnish with minced green onions, lemon or lime slices, and sliced hot peppers or pepper sauce, if desired.

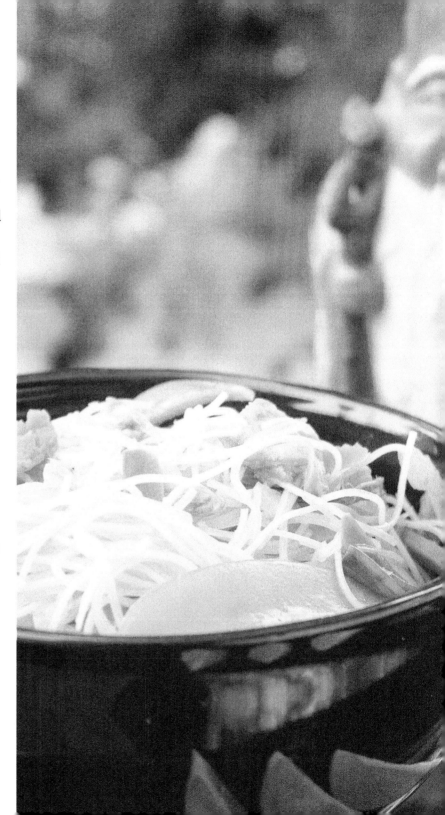

Prize Winning Cabbage & Carrots
Serves 4

With a head of cabbage, a Fresno pepper plant bursting with peppers on my deck, a carton of chicken broth, an onion and two lonely carrots, I created a really tasty vegetable side dish. I submitted the original version of this recipe to a medical center's Healthy Recipe Contest, and won the first prize of $100. So I can honestly claim this dish as a prize-winning recipe.

Ingredients

2 carrots, waffle cut or julienned

1 small head cabbage, thinly sliced

1 medium yellow onion, thinly sliced then quartered

1½ cups not-chicken or vegetable broth

1-2 whole red Fresno (or red jalapeño or other hot pepper)

1-3 teaspoons olive oil (depends on the stickiness of your cooking pot – I use cast iron)

Salt and pepper to taste

Instructions

- Put olive oil in large skillet and heat over medium. When oil is hot, add the sliced onions. Sauté onions for 1-2 minutes or until onions are soft.
- Add the thinly sliced cabbage and stir to mix everything up nicely. Sauté for about 2-3 minutes until some of the cabbage is lightly browned.
- Add the carrots and broth, stirring to coat cabbage mixture evenly; cover pan.
- Let cabbage steam/simmer for about six minutes. Cut your red pepper into 8-10 lengthwise slivers, removing the seeds to reduce the heat. Place sliced peppers in the pan and stir.
- Replace top and cook another 6-10 minutes until cabbage is done to your liking.
- Top with a sprinkle of balsamic or red wine vinegar and enjoy!

Stir Fried Tofu in Vegan Oyster Sauce

Serves 2-3

Tofu is a rich source of vegan protein, low in calories and high in calcium, Omega-3 fats, selenium, magnesium, iron and protein. Look for the tofu with calcium sulfate on the list of ingredients for a boost to your daily calcium intake.

Ingredients

1 small (4 oz) can mushrooms

¼ cup bamboo shoots, sliced

1 package firm organic non-GMO tofu, cut into 1" cubes

½ teaspoon salt

2 Tablespoons vegan oyster sauce

1½ teaspoons arrowroot powder mixed with 2 Tablespoons of water

½ teaspoon agave nectar

Peanut oil

2 green onions, cut into 1" pieces

Instructions

- Heat 1 Tablespoon peanut oil in wok or large skillet and stir fry mushrooms and bamboo shoots over high heat about 1 minute. Sprinkle with 2 Tablespoons of water. Cook another 10 seconds or so then remove ingredients and liquid from wok.
- Heat 2 Tablespoons oil in wok and add the cut tofu. Stir fry until slightly crisped.
- Add ½ teaspoon salt and 1 Tablespoon of water. Pour in the oyster sauce, then add the mushrooms and bamboo shoots.
- Stir gently to combine ingredients. Add cornstarch mixture and cook until slightly thickened.
- Garnish with green onion, and serve immediately with rice.

New Orleans Style Red Beans & Rice
Makes 8 Servings

I love red beans and rice, but as a vegan I faced the dilemma of achieving the meaty flavor, spicy broth and rich warm aroma without meat. After quite a bit of trial and error... a winner! Try the andouille sausage style seitan recipe here - it's fabulous.

Ingredients

1 quart carton vegetable broth
7 cups water
2 Tablespoons not-chicken concentrate
2 onions, chopped
1 green bell pepper, chopped
3 celery stalks, chopped
5 cloves garlic, minced
2 bay leaves
1 pound of dried small red or kidney beans
1½ teaspoons dried thyme leaves
¼ teaspoon powdered allspice
1 teaspoon vegan Worcestershire sauce
1 teaspoon agave nectar
½ teaspoon ancho chili powder
2 pinches baking soda
6 dried pequin pepper pods
½ teaspoon black pepper
1½ to 2 packets Goya Ham flavored seasoning
½ teaspoon smoked salt (optional)
1 package commercial vegan or homemade Andouille style vegan sausage (page 150)

Instructions

- Put broth and water in large pot over low heat. While it's heating up, clean the beans - removing any broken or shriveled beans and debris. Rinse beans thoroughly in colander, then add to pot.

- Add chopped onion, bell pepper, celery, and garlic.

- Add the remaining spices and herbs (except for the smoked salt in case you decide it's salty enough without it).

- Slow simmer over low heat for about 3½ hours, stirring a few times every hour.

- Taste and adjust salt and pepper. Smash a few beans against the side of the pot with back of spoon; stir and continue to cook another 20 minutes.

- Diagonally slice your vegan sausages about ¼" thick; brown them in a little oil and set aside.

- Remove pot from burner and let sit, covered, for another 15 minutes before serving over traditional white rice, quinoa or millet.

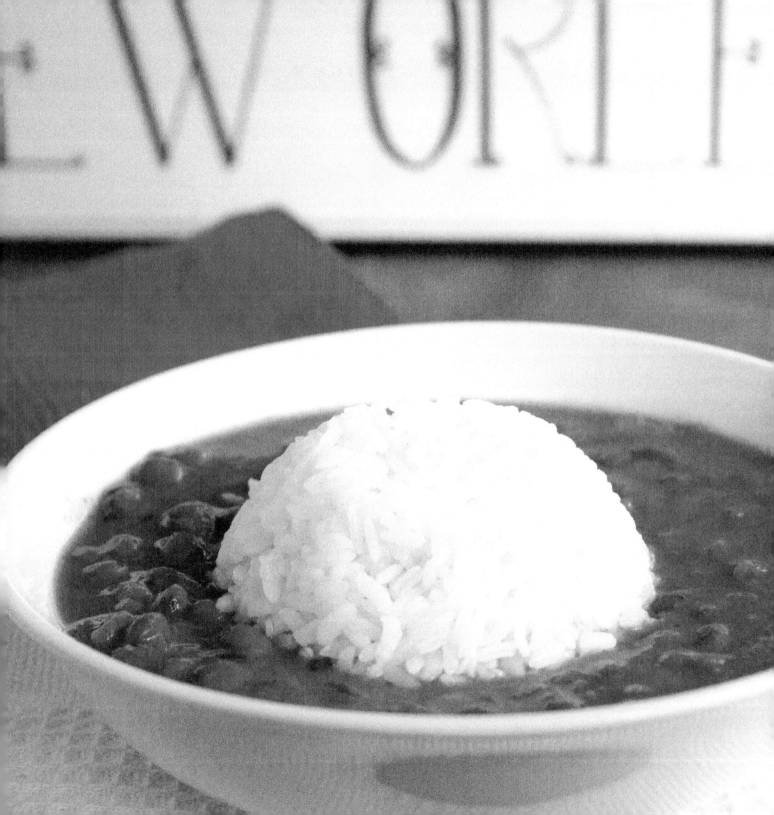

Quinoa Rotelle Mac and Cheese
Serves 4-6

My favorite pasta these days is rotelle made out of quinoa. The nooks and crannies of the spirals really help the sauces hold onto the pasta, so every bite has lots of flavor and saucy goodness.

Ingredients

8 oz box of quinoa rotelle
1 teaspoon olive oil
¼ cup vegan butter
1 large shallot, minced
1 clove garlic, minced
3 Tablespoons unbleached flour
⅓ cup nutritional yeast (more or less to taste)
1 carton plain soy creamer (12 oz)
½ teaspoon Himalayan pink salt
⅛ teaspoon turmeric
1 teaspoon spicy brown mustard
1 Tablespoon chili sauce
⅛ teaspoon cayenne
¼ teaspoon fresh ground black pepper
1 teaspoon agave nectar
Paprika for garnish

Instructions

- Boil 8 cups water in pot; add bit of salt and olive oil. Once water is boiling, cook pasta according to package directions. Drain into a bowl (retaining the cooking water), and set pasta aside.
- In a nonstick sauce pan, melt the vegan butter over medium heat. Add the garlic and shallot. Cook, stirring frequently about 1 minute. Slowly add in the flour, stirring to blend until smooth. Let cook, stirring frequently, until flour becomes a light toasty brown.
- Reduce heat to low, then add in the soy creamer, nutritional yeast, salt, cayenne, turmeric, mustard, agave and chili sauce. Let mixture cook until thickened but still pourable (cheese sauce).
- Taste and adjust salt if needed. Sprinkle with fresh ground black pepper and paprika. Serve hot.

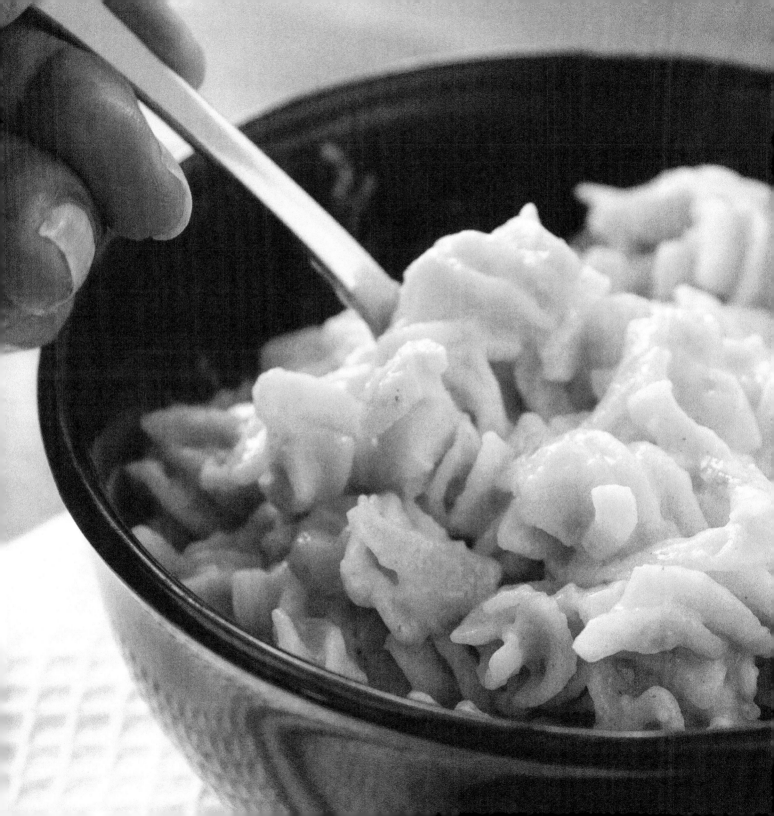

Black Bean Lasagna
Serves 8-10

This recipe takes time to make, so plan ahead. The spices and seasonings replace my original omni recipe for lasagna, providing a close imitation to the hot Italian sausage sauce I used before going vegan.

Ingredients

12 lasagna noodles
1 recipe tofu ricotta (below)
8 oz vegan Mozzarella style strips
3 Tablespoons fresh basil, chopped fine
3 Tablespoons olive oil
1 10 oz package frozen chopped spinach, thawed and pressed to remove excess water

Black Bean Sauce

3 cups precooked or canned black beans
1 teaspoon dried oregano leaves
1 teaspoon granulated sugar
1 teaspoon garlic powder
1 teaspoon dried thyme leaves
1 teaspoon ground black pepper
½ teaspoon red pepper flakes
½ teaspoon ground fennel
1 28 oz can San Marzano style chopped tomatoes (with juice)
1 teaspoon granulated onion powder
4 cloves garlic, minced
½ teaspoon paprika

1 yellow onion, minced (between 1½ to 2 cups)
½ green bell pepper, minced (about ⅔ cup)
½ cup red wine
1 teaspoon olive oil
2 teaspoons garlic salt

Tofu Ricotta

¼ cup raw cashews, finely ground
1 14 oz carton firm or extra-firm tofu, frozen, thawed and pressed to remove extra water
¼ cup good quality nutritional yeast
3 Tablespoons olive oil
1 teaspoon Himalayan pink salt (or to taste)

Instructions

• Place 1 teaspoon olive oil in non-stick skillet. When heated, add the onion, garlic and bell pepper and sauté over med-low heat until translucent (about 3 minutes).

• Combine onion mixture with bean mixture in a large sauce pan. Add ½ cup red wine or water, stir, and bring to a boil. Reduce heat to low and simmer, partially covered, for about 20-30 minutes to thicken.

- Bring large pot of salted water to boil and cook lasagna noodles according to package directions. Remove from heat about 3 minutes before fully cooked. Drain, rinse in cold water, and set aside.

- Prepare your ricotta mixture. In a good sized bowl, place the prepared tofu ricotta, ¾ of the mozzarella shreds, spinach, parsley, basil, salt and pepper, and mix together thoroughly. Set aside.

To assemble the lasagna:

- Spread 1½ cups of the thickened sauce in bottom of a 9x13" baking pan. Place 3 of the noodles lengthwise, then top them with ⅓ of the cheese/spinach mixture, spreading so that it is evenly distributed.

- Add a layer of noodles, and another 1 to 1½ cups of sauce, then top with the cheese/spinach mixture, and repeat until last layer of noodles. Add remaining sauce on top of noodles and sprinkle with reserved mozzarella strips.

- Cover with foil and bake at 375 degrees for 30-35 minutes. Remove foil and cook another 10-15 minutes to brown slightly.

- Allow dish to "set" out to cool for approximately 20 minutes before slicing into squares to serve.

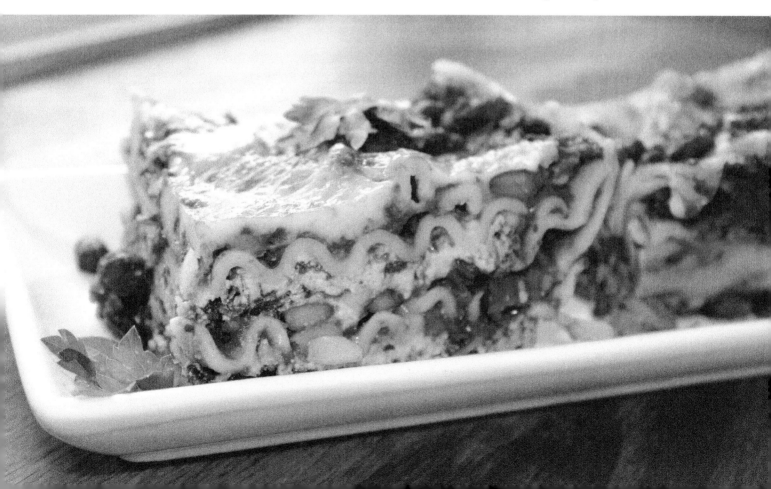

Tasty Seasoned Chickpeas
Makes 6 Cups

I make a pot of these every two weeks or so and use them for roasted chickpea snacks, in soup and salad recipes, or hummus. Cooking in a pressure cooker eliminates the need for presoaking and provides almost instant gratification. If you don't have a pressure cooker, just follow these directions.

Ingredients

2 cups dried chickpeas

6 cups water

2 peeled carrots, cut into thirds

2 shallots (not green onions, the brown oniony garlicky shallots)

12 black peppercorns

2 stalks celery, trimmed and cut into thirds

3 stems fresh thyme

1 bay leaf

1 piece cheesecloth

½ herbal vegetable bouillon cube

½ teaspoon sea salt

Instructions

- Place rinsed and cleaned chickpeas into a bowl and cover with water 1" past fill line. Let soak 10-12 hours/overnight.
- In the morning, drain and rinse chickpeas. Put into pot and add water.
- Tie herbs, vegetables, peppercorns, and bay leaf up in cheesecloth and place on top of chickpeas.
- Let mixture come to a boil, then lower heat, stir, and simmer uncovered for 45-60 minutes or until tender, but not mushy. Stir occasionally, adding additional water if needed to keep peas from sticking.
- Add ½ teaspoon sea salt about 45 minutes into cooking. Avoid adding salt too early as it toughens beans and chickpeas.
- When done, taste and adjust seasonings.

Quick Vegetable and Bean Soup
Makes 6 Servings

A little of this, a little of that, ended up with a really tasty soup. Served it with fresh cornbread. Nobody complained. Win.

Ingredients

2 Tablespoons olive oil
1 can organic crushed fire roasted tomatoes
3 cloves garlic, minced (1 heaping tablespoon)
2 stalks celery
½ large onion
1 leek, bottom white part only, cut into quarters and sliced fine
1 vegetable bouillon with herbs cube
2 bags organic mixed vegetables
3 quarts vegetable stock (low sodium or home made)
2 quarts water
3 large red potatoes, scrubbed and diced
½ red bell pepper, minced
2 teaspoons dried basil leaves
2 teaspoons ground black pepper
1 teaspoon Kosher salt
2 Tablespoons nutritional yeast
½ cup rinsed but uncooked quinoa
1 can organic Great Northern beans, drained

Instructions

- Add olive oil to large stock pot. Heat over medium. Add celery, onion, garlic and leeks and sauté until onion is translucent.
- Stir in can of tomatoes, basil, pepper and salt. Let simmer 2-3 minutes.
- Add vegetable stock, vegetable cube and half the water. Stir and let simmer 10 minutes
- Add remaining ingredients, cover pot and let soup simmer for 40 minutes.
- Serve with side salad and/or cornbread or toasted whole grain bread.

Vegan Sausage & Mushroom Pizza
Serves 3-4

Use a package of ready-to-go pizza dough or a prepared pizza crust to make it even easier. Naan or other flat bread also makes a great pizza crust. Add your favorite vegetable toppings, such as sun dried tomatoes, roasted garlic, or artichoke hearts. Makes one 12-14" round pizza.

Ingredients

1 package pizza crust dough or one prepared crust
1 cup each red, yellow, and orange pepper slices
½ large red onion, sliced thin and halved
½ 8 oz package sliced mushrooms
2 teaspoons olive oil
2 cups fresh organic baby spinach leaves
2 medium Roma tomatoes, sliced thin
⅓ cup sliced olives
½ cup chopped vegan breakfast or Italian sausage

Cheezy Tomato Pizza Sauce
1 15 oz can organic tomato sauce
2-3 Tablespoons chopped fresh basil
1 teaspoon agave nectar
1 teaspoon garlic salt
½ teaspoon granulated onion
½ teaspoon fresh ground black pepper
½ teaspoon dried oregano leaves
¼ teaspoon Italian seasoning
½ cup raw cashews soaked in ½ cup water for 30 minutes, drained
1½ Tablespoons nutritional yeast flakes

Instructions

• Place drained cashews and all other sauce ingredients in blender and puree until smooth; taste and adjust seasonings as needed.

• Preheat oven to 450 degrees. Heat olive oil in large non-stick skillet over medium heat. Add onions and pepper, and sauté until soft about 5 minutes. Add mushrooms and continue cooking another two minutes or until mushrooms are softened but not mushy.

• Stretch out dough to fit your pizza pan, or place prepared crust/flat bread on baking tray. Use about half the cheezy tomato sauce, adding more if desired. Top with spinach leaves, sautéed vegetables, olives and vegan sausage.

• Bake for about 15 minutes, then slide pizza off pan directly onto oven rack and bake another 5-8 minutes for additional crispiness.

• Cut into 6-8 slices and serve with vegan Parmesan, chopped fresh garlic, and red pepper flakes for toppings.

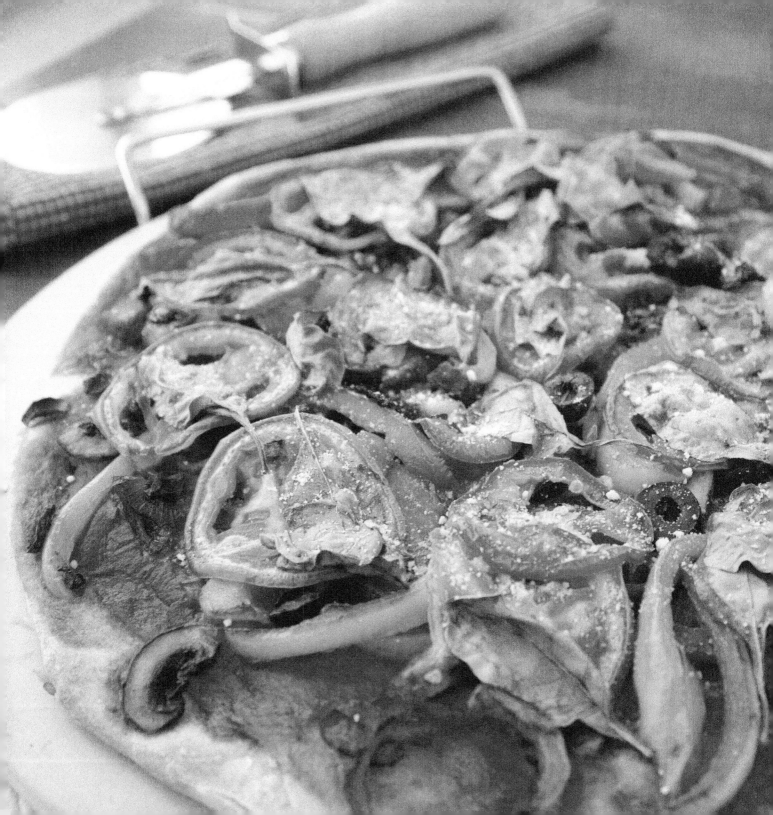

"Beef" Barley Soup with 'Shrooms
Serves 8

High protein, satisfying soup for cold fall and winter months. Travels well, so it's great to pack in thermal jugs for lunches at work or school.

Ingredients

2 Tablespoons vegetable oil

1 medium onion, diced

2 large carrots, chopped

12 oz package cremini mushrooms, sliced thin

½ teaspoon dried thyme leaves (or 2 teaspoons minced fresh thyme)

1-2 Roma tomatoes, diced (about ½ cup)

4 cups hot water

4 teaspoons not-beef seasoning paste

1 package vegan "beef" tips, cut into bite-sized pieces

½ cup pearl barley

¼ cup minced fresh parsley leaves

Himalayan pink salt and fresh ground black pepper to taste

Instructions

• Heat oil over medium high heat in a large soup pot. Add onion and carrots, and sauté until translucent (about 3-4 minutes)

• Add sliced mushrooms and sauté until soft. At this point most of the liquid from vegetables should be evaporated.

• Add thyme and tomatoes, not-beef paste, "beef" tips, and barley.

• Bring to a boil, then reduce heat to low and simmer until barley is tender - about 45 minutes.

• Stir in parsley and adjust seasonings to taste.

Broccoli in Shallot and Orange Butter
Makes 6 Servings

This was one of my favorite recipes often prepared for family gatherings by my Uncle Bill, who worked as a professional chef for decades. In my version the dairy butter is replaced with vegan butter, but other than that the recipe is exactly the same as he made it for decades.

Ingredients

3 pounds broccoli crowns

1 teaspoon salt

½ cup fresh organic orange juice

1½ sticks (¾ cup) vegan butter

⅓ cup minced shallot

1½ Tablespoons organic orange peel, julienned (orange skin only)

Pinch of sea or pink salt

Instructions

- Put on large pot of water to boil. Add a teaspoon or so of salt.
- Cut broccoli into serving-size florets, then cook in boiling salted water until tender crisp (about 5 minutes).
- Drain pot in colander and run under cold tap to immediately stop broccoli from cooking further. Pat dry with paper towels.
- Simmer orange juice in a small, heavy-bottomed sauce pan until reduced slightly (8-10 minutes).
- Melt butter in a large heavy skillet over low heat, then add minced shallot and orange peel. Cover and cook until shallots are tender, stirring occasionally (about 6-8 minutes).
- Mix in reduced orange juice, pinch of salt and broccoli. Raise heat to medium and toss broccoli in sauce for a few minutes until heated through and thoroughly coated.

Chickpea Mock Chicken Salad
Makes 4-6 Servings

This recipe is created from the Tasty Seasoned Chickpeas, but if in a pinch, just open a can. You can make four salads, or about six sandwiches per recipe. Use a potato masher or a pastry blender to mash the chickpeas into lumpy smoothness, removing any skins that you can see. If making sandwiches, try toasting the bread first, as it helps prevent sogginess.

Ingredients

½ cup minced red onion (or 1 Tablespoon dried onion flakes)

2 cups Tasty Seasoned Chickpeas (or 1 16 oz can, rinsed and drained thoroughly)

2 green onions, minced (white and green top)

⅓ to ½ cup vegan mayo (as you like it)

4 gherkin pickles, minced

½ teaspoon fresh ground black pepper

3 stalks celery, chopped fine

1 carrot, peeled and grated (about ½ cup)

¼ teaspoon garlic powder

¼ teaspoon sea salt

1 teaspoon vegan Worcestershire sauce

Instructions

• Mix all ingredients together.

• Refrigerate for 30 minutes or more to allow flavors to blend.

• For variety, add 1 cup red seedless organic grapes, which have been cut in half (as pictured)

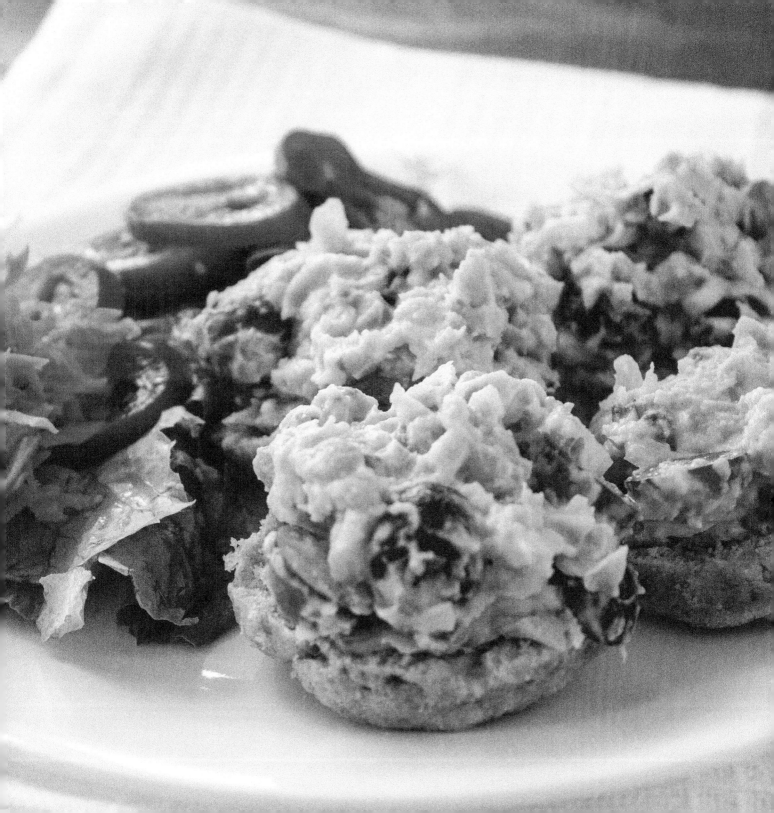

Vegan Spaghettini Carbonara
Serves 4

This simple and traditional Italian pasta dish basically translates to "bacon and egg pasta". Commercially available coconut bacon or vegan bacon-flavored soy bits fill in nicely; The Vegg® creates a rich egg-yolk like palate sensation and taste.

Ingredients

1 lb. spaghettini, fettuccine, or tagliatelle pasta

1 Tablespoon The Vegg® powder

2 cups pasta cooking water

½ teaspoon not-chicken seasoning paste

1 Tablespoon nutritional yeast flakes

¼ teaspoon sea salt

½ teaspoon black pepper

3-4 Tablespoons olive oil

2 Tablespoons garlic, chopped fine

1 teaspoon red pepper flakes

2 Tablespoons vegan butter

⅓ cup vegan bacon bits (coconut bacon works well too)

½ cup or more chopped fresh flat-leaf Italian parsley (optional)

Fresh ground black pepper and salt to taste

Instructions

- Cook pasta in salted boiling water per instructions to al dente (still slightly firm), usually about 7-8 minutes. Drain cooking water into a bowl (retaining 2 cups or more for your sauce), and set pasta aside.
- Put 2 cups of somewhat cooled pasta cooking water, seasoning paste, nutritional yeast flakes, black pepper, sea salt, and The Vegg® powder into blender. Blend for 15-20 seconds.
- Heat a large skillet over low heat. Add the olive oil, red pepper flakes and garlic and cook about 2 minutes, stirring frequently.
- Pour in The Vegg® mixture and vegan butter, and let simmer until slightly thickened, about 4-5 minutes.

- Add drained pasta to skillet and toss well to evenly coat the spaghetti. Toss in half or more of your vegan bacon bits and stir again.
- Turn off heat and taste – add more salt and pepper if needed. Continue tossing pasta until it absorbs the sauce (1-2 minutes).
- Garnish with the rest of your bacon bits. Sprinkle with vegan Parmesan and chopped parsley if desired.

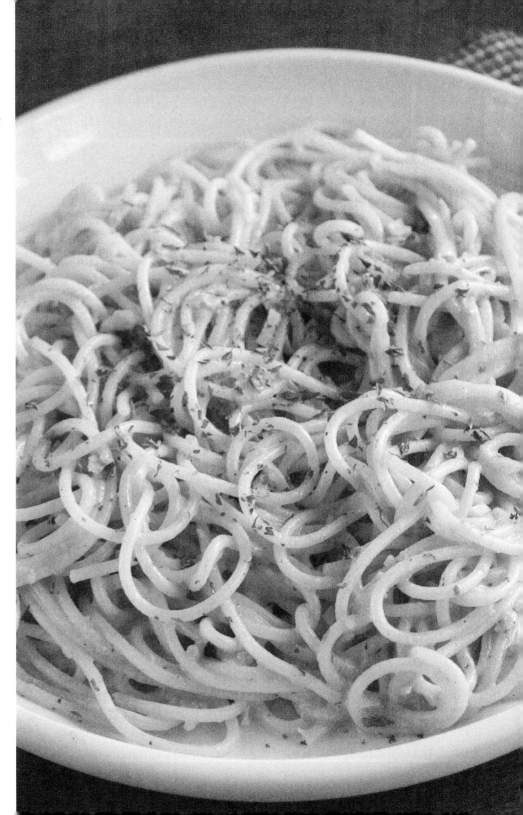

Red Potatoes Roasted with Garlic & Rosemary
Serves 4-6

Believe it or not, my daughter came up with this idea a few years ago when our three scrawny rosemary bushes suddenly decided to grow. To tell you the truth, she was putting rosemary on any and everything... it got kinda ridiculous. Great plain, with ketchup or Parmesan cheeze.

Ingredients

4-5 good-sized red potatoes, cut into cube or wedge shapes

4 Tablespoons olive oil

4-5 cloves garlic, chopped

2 Tablespoons minced fresh rosemary (leaves only)

1 Tablespoon fresh parsley, minced

2 teaspoons seasoning salt

1½ teaspoons fresh ground black pepper

Instructions

• Preheat oven to 425 degrees.

• Use one Tablespoon of the olive oil to coat a rimmed baking sheet. Place pan in the oven until hot (about 5 minutes).

• While pan heats, place potato cubes/wedges, remaining olive oil, chopped garlic, rosemary, parsley, seasoning salt and ground pepper in a plastic bag. Close bag and shake vigorously to distribute oil and seasonings evenly onto potatoes.

• Remove seasoned potatoes from bag and put on hot baking sheet in a single layer.

• Bake for about 25 minutes, then flip to other side and continue baking another 20-25 minutes. Potatoes should be golden brown and lightly crispy all over.

Gingered Baby Carrots
Serves 5-6

Dieters, children, party goers – everyone eats baby carrots. This recipe is a tasty side dish with the non-traditional zing of fresh ginger, tempered with the buttery sweetness of brown sugar. To peel the ginger before grating, hold a paring knife against ginger root and gently scrape the paper thin skin off.

Ingredients

1½ lb bag of baby carrots

¾ cup not-chicken broth

4 Tablespoons (½ stick) vegan butter

1½ Tablespoons dark brown sugar

2 Tablespoons grated fresh ginger

1 Tablespoon chopped fresh parsley leaves

Instructions

• Place carrots, butter, brown sugar and grated ginger in a heavy bottomed saucepan. Cover the pan and cook over medium heat until the carrots are tender-crisp (about 10 minutes).

• Remove the lid and cook over medium-high heat, stirring occasionally, for about 5 minutes or until liquid reduces to a syrup that coats the carrots.

• Transfer to a serving bowl and toss with the parsley.

Hoppin' John
Serves 8

Every New Year's, somebody in my Dad's family would make a black eyed pea and rice dish called Hoppin' John. I don't know who John is or why he was hoppin', but I do know this was one of my favorite things to eat growing up. The problem is it used a lot of bacon, which served as the flavoring source. Here's the flavorful remake of one of my family's traditional dishes.

Ingredients

1 pound of dried black-eyed peas
4 Tablespoons Magic Vegan Bacon grease
1½ cups minced onion
½ cup green bell pepper, minced
½ cup celery, minced
2 cartons (8 cups) vegetable or not-chicken broth
2 cups water
3 Tablespoons not-chicken seasoning base
2 cloves garlic, minced
¼ teaspoon cayenne pepper
1 teaspoon dried thyme leaves
1 bay leaf
1/8 teaspoon dried rosemary
1 teaspoon smoked salt flakes
1 Tablespoon Bac-Uns Vegetarian bits
1 teaspoon smoked paprika
½ teaspoon smoked or regular pepper
2 cups uncooked long-grain white rice
¾ cup chopped green onions

Instructions

- Clean and pick the black eyed peas, and soak them for at least 5 hours in water. Drain and rinse.
- Put Magic Bacon Grease into a large pot, and over medium heat sauté the onion, bell pepper and celery until onion is transparent.
- Add your broth, water, and seasoning base and Bac-Un bits, and bring pot to a boil.
- Add minced garlic, bay leaf, rosemary, thyme, salt, pepper, and cayenne. Stir well.
- Add the drained and rinsed black eyed peas. Partially cover the pot (you want some evaporation here), and slow-simmer for about 90 minutes.
- Add 2 cups uncooked long-grain rice and stir well. Cover pot and continue cooking for 20 minutes. Turn off stove and let pot sit on hot burner for an additional 10-15 minutes to steam and fluff the rice.
- Remove top, and stir in chopped green onions. If desired sprinkle on and stir in a teaspoon or so of Bac-Un bits for an extra flavor boost.

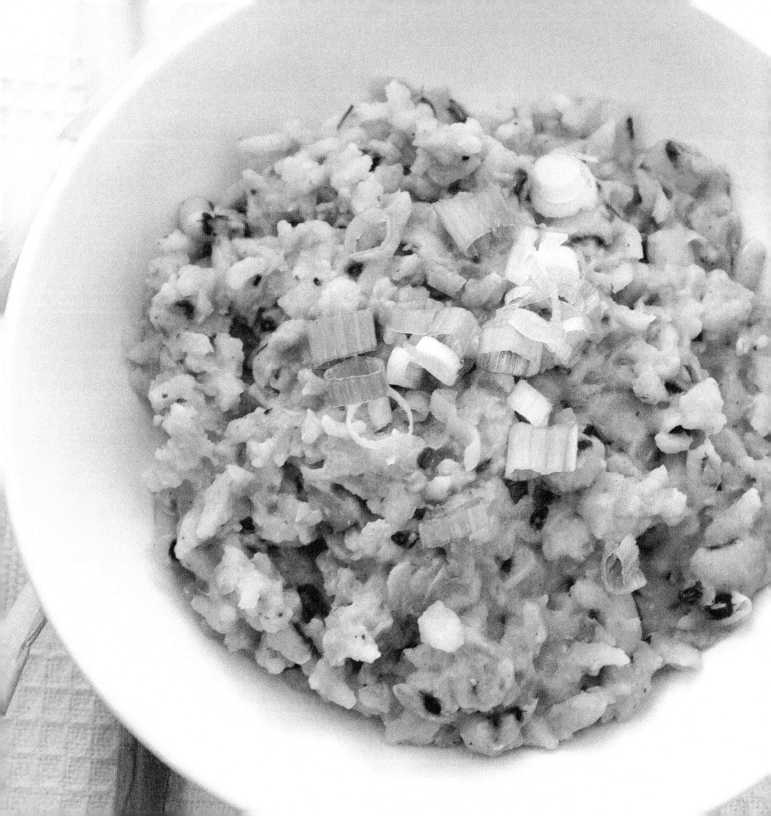

Peppery Sweet Potatoes and Fresh Thyme
Serves 4

Make these as "peppery" as you like by adding more or less red pepper flakes.

Ingredients

4 medium sweet potatoes

3 Tablespoons olive oil

4 cloves garlic, minced

⅓ cup fresh thyme leaves

½ teaspoon kosher salt

½ teaspoon red pepper flakes

‡ Alternative Seasoning Combinations

Thyme, chili powder, garlic powder, sea salt

Garlic powder, turmeric, sea salt

Cinnamon, paprika, sea salt

Nutmeg, cinnamon, sea salt

Brown sugar, cinnamon, sea salt

Black pepper, sea salt, paprika

Instructions

- Preheat oven to 450 degrees.
- Spray 9x13" baking dish with non-stick spray.
- In large mixing bowl, combine all ingredients and toss to coat potatoes thoroughly.
- Arrange seasoned potato slices in a single layer in prepared baking dish.
- Roast potatoes in oven under cooked through and lightly browned, about 45 minutes.
- Best served warm.

Fusilli Pasta Salad With Broccoli
Makes 6-8 Servings

Great take-along for office or family potlucks, plus it's good to keep around for warm days when light food made without the oven is called for. Who doesn't like a good pasta salad? If you like spicy, increase the red pepper flakes.

Ingredients

2-3 broccoli crowns, cut into bite-sized florets (about 7 cups total)

¼ cup lemon juice

½ teaspoon grated lemon zest

1 clove garlic, minced

½ teaspoon red pepper flakes

½ cup extra virgin olive oil

1 lb quinoa or plain white fusilli or farfalle pasta

20 large pitted kalamata olives, chopped

15 large fresh basil leaves, sliced thin

Instructions

- Bring 4 quarts of water to boil in a large pot over high heat. Also bring several quarts of water to boil in a large saucepan. Add salt to taste to both.
- Add broccoli florets to saucepan and cook until tender-crisp, about 2 minutes. Drain into colander and cool to room temperature.
- Whisk together lemon juice and lemon zest, the garlic, ¾ teaspoon of sea salt, and red pepper flakes in a large bowl. Slowly pour in the oil and whisk until smooth.
- Add pasta to boiling, salted water. Cook until pasta is al dente according to package directions. Drain and return to pot.
- Whisk your dressing again if it has separated, then add the red peppers, broccoli, olives and basil; mix thoroughly.
- Allow pasta salad to cool to room temp, then taste and adjust seasonings.

Potato and Mushroom Soup
Serves 4

This mild soup is unbelievably simple to make. Just a few ingredients come together to make a surprisingly rich, creamy and filling main course soup. I prefer cashew milk here, but your favorite plant milk should work fine. Serve with crusty sourdough bread and a side salad.

Ingredients

¼ cup vegan butter

1½ pounds Yukon gold potatoes, peeled and diced

1 large onion, diced

2 Tablespoons vegan butter or olive oil

1 lb cremini or white mushrooms

Salt and fresh ground black pepper to taste

1 quart carton vegetable broth

1 cup soy or almond milk

Fresh thyme and parsley leaves

Instructions

- Place vegan butter in large heavy-bottomed saucepan over medium heat. Once melted, add potatoes and onions, salt and pepper.
- Reduce heat to low, cover pan, and let vegetables simmer in their own juices for a few minutes. Add a Tablespoon or two of the stock to make sure they stay moist.
- Bring stock to a boil in small pot. Once vegetables are tender, add boiling stock to saucepan and simmer for 10 minutes, or until veggies are tender.
- Blend right in the pot using a stick blender, and let cook another 5 minutes.
- Sauté sliced mushrooms in vegan butter or olive oil in non-stick frying pan until browned. Add chopped parsley and thyme and stir well.
- Add the plant milk to potatoes and stir in half the sautéed mushrooms.
- Season to taste and garnish with remaining sautéed mushrooms.

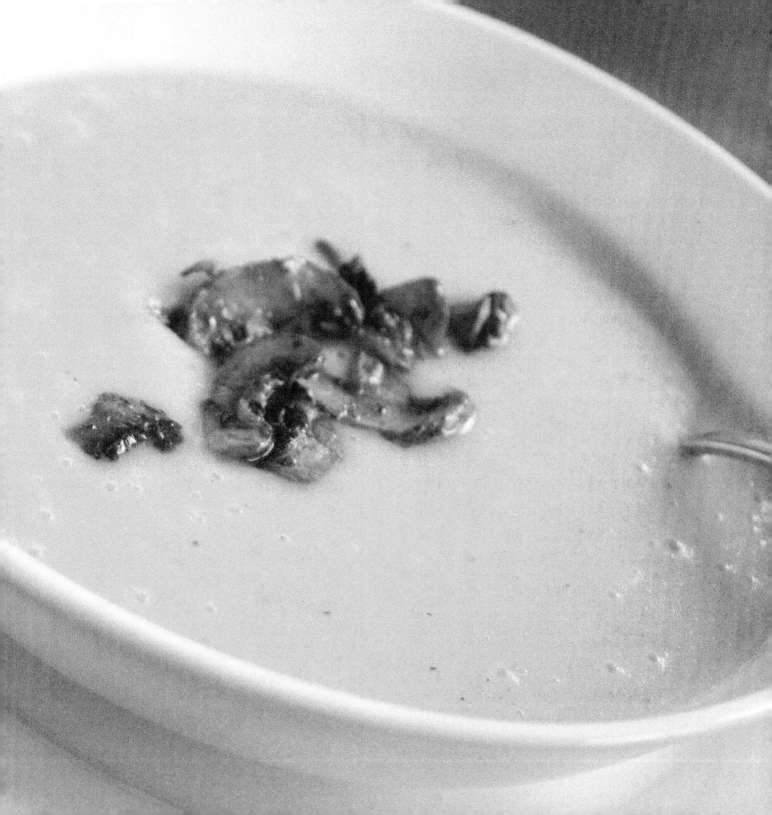

Spicy Black Beans in Pressure Cooker
Serves 8-10

I love making my black beans with a pressure cooker, which helps cut down on cooking time and eliminates the need for presoaking. That essentially means that no advance planning is required if I decide at 3:00 pm that I'd love black beans for dinner at 6:00 pm.

Ingredients

1 pound black beans, cleaned and rinsed

1 Tablespoon olive oil

1 large onion, chopped (about 2 cups)

1 large green bell pepper, chopped small

3-4 cloves garlic, minced

1 teaspoon ground cumin

2 Tablespoons Ancho chili powder

1 jalapeño pepper, seeds removed and minced

1 8 oz can salade de chile fresco tomato sauce

8 cups water

3 not-chicken bouillon cubes

1½ teaspoons dried oregano leaves

1 3" piece Kombu seaweed

2 Tablespoons agave nectar

2-3 Tablespoons red wine vinegar

1 teaspoon Himalayan pink salt (or to taste)

Instructions

• Place first 13 ingredients into pressure cooker and stir to mix. Add top to pressure cooker and heat over medium-high heat until pressure builds and pressure indicator starts rocking steadily.

• Reduce heat to low and simmer along for 45 minutes. Remove pressure cooker from heat and let cool about 20 minutes or until pressure releases.

• Stir in agave and vinegar; taste and adjust salt and pepper as required, adding Himalayan pink salt and more vinegar if necessary.

• Serve with Mexicali Red Rice (page 60), tortillas, pico de gallo, vegan cheese, or vegan sour cream. Or use them for any recipe which uses black beans.

Black Bean & Sweet Potato Soup
Serves 4

This is another creation inspired by my "throw it in a pot and sit down" method of meal preparation. With leftover black beans, a huge sweet potato lurking on the counter, and a "here, try this" bag of Ancient Grains in my freezer, this really delicious and filling recipe was truly an accident.

Ingredients

2 cups previous prepared Spicy Black Beans

¼ teaspoon celery seeds

3 Tablespoons dried onion flakes

1 carton (quart) vegetable broth

1 vegetable bouillon cube

1 Tablespoon not-chicken seasoning base

½ teaspoon garlic powder

1 large sweet potato, peeled and diced (about 4 cups)

1 package Engine 2 brand Ancient Grains blend

1 cup water

1 teaspoon fresh ground black pepper

1 teaspoon kosher salt

12 organic grape tomatoes, cut in half

Instructions

• Put all ingredients into a large pot and let it simmer, uncovered, until potatoes are soft (about 30 minutes.

• Watch water level, adding more as needed if it gets too thick.

Sweet Potato Fries
Serves 4

I've been eating sweet potato fries since I was old enough to feed myself. My grand wasn't into store bought food, and didn't think very highly of greasy French fries either. I still can't get the crunch that she did, but this comes close. The tricks to success? #1 don't crowd the baking sheet - give each fry space on all sides; #2 bake only one pan at a time right in the center of the oven; and #3 cut your sweet potatoes as uniformly as possible for even cooking.

Ingredients

4 medium sized sweet potatoes (about 3 pounds)

3 Tablespoons olive or canola oil

1 Tablespoon paprika

1 Tablespoon chili powder

1 teaspoon cayenne

1½ teaspoons garlic powder

Non-stick spray

Instructions

- Preheat oven to 425 degrees. Put spices in a large plastic or paper bag. Shake spices to mix them together.
- Cut sweet potatoes into ½" thick French fry shapes. You can peel them first or just scrub the skins really well with a vegetable brush and dry them off with paper towels.
- Dump cut potatoes into large bowl and coat lightly with oil. Mix around to coat fries evenly with the oil.
- Transfer oiled potatoes to bag with seasoning. Toss them in the bag for about 30 seconds to ensure that each fry is uniformly covered with spices.
- Arrange fries on baking sheets coated with non-stick spray, leaving at least ¼" space around each fry.
- Place baking sheets in oven and cook fries for about 15 minutes. Flip them over using metal spatula, and continue baking for another 10-12 minutes, or until fries are crispy, brown and caramelized on the edges.

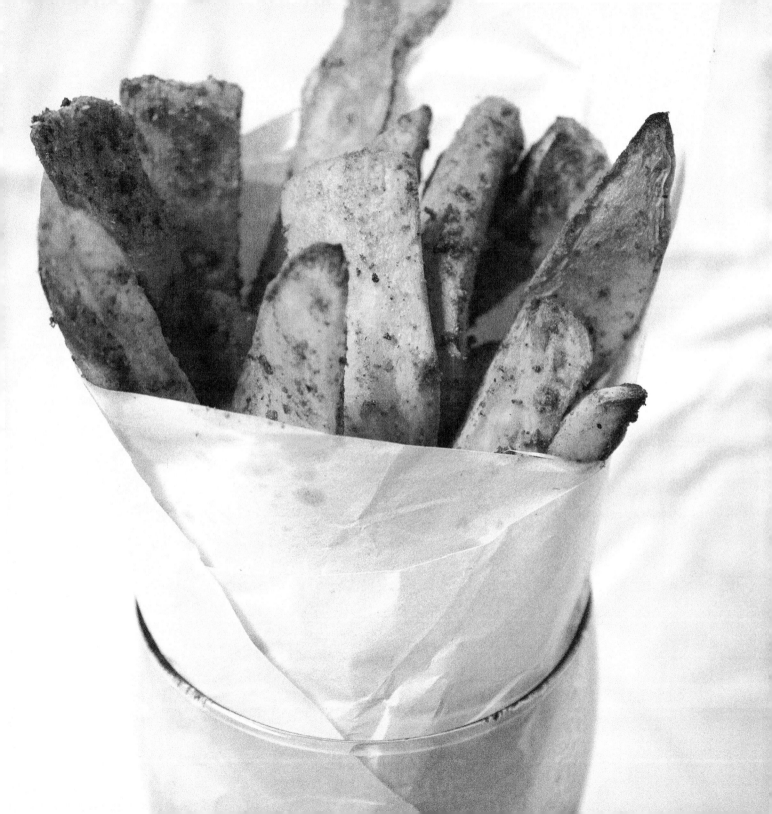

Navy Bean Crock Pot Soup
Serves 8

Another recipe from the files that my Grand used to make all the time, though use of a crock pot is my way of getting the job done. I eliminated the salt pork that she used for seasoning and replaced it with not-chicken broth.

Ingredients

1 16 oz bag of dried navy beans, sorted and rinsed

1 cup carrots, chopped fine

1 cup minced celery, including leaves

½ cup minced onion

8 cups water

2 not-chicken bouillon cubes

1 cup vegetable juice cocktail

¼ teaspoon crushed red pepper flakes

Instructions

- Combine all ingredients in 4 quart crock pot. Stir to mix well.
- Cover and cook over low heat all day (for at least 8 hours).
- Delicious served with corn bread.

Wilted Spinach Salad
Serves 2-3

Wilted spinach salads are usually served with hot bacon grease - but we aren't doing saturated animal fat, remember? Try this lighter, but still tasty version of a classic.

Ingredients

1 pound fresh baby spinach leaves

3 Tablespoons olive or walnut oil

⅓ cup finely chopped green onions

1 clove garlic, minced

1 Tablespoon raw apple cider vinegar

Salt and fresh ground black pepper to taste

Fresh grated nutmeg

Instructions

- Wash and drain spinach thoroughly, remove coarse stems.
- Heat oil in large sauté pan; add green onions and garlic. Cook, stirring until green onions are soft (about 4 minutes).
- Add spinach, vinegar, salt, pepper and a few gratings of nutmeg.
- Cook and stir another minute or two, until spinach is heated through (it should look shiny and be slightly wilted).

Basic Chicken-Style Seitan
Makes 1¼ Pounds

Seitan is a 100% vegan protein supplement used in most ways as you did in your meat-eating days. Also known as "wheat meat," seitan provides the same protein as beef without any of the saturated fat or cholesterol, and less than half the calories. Recipes for creating many different flavors of seitan follow, along with flavorful family friendly dishes which use them.

Ingredients

2 Tablespoons vegetarian not-chicken base

6 cups water

2 green onions

1 cup vital wheat gluten

2 Tablespoons chickpea flour

1 Tablespoon nutritional yeast

½ teaspoon onion powder

½ teaspoon garlic powder

½ teaspoon poultry seasoning

¼ teaspoon sea salt

¼ teaspoon black pepper

¾ cup water or vegetable broth

1 Tablespoon vegetable oil

Instructions

- Add the vegetarian not-chicken seasoning and green onions to the water. Alternatively, use vegetable stock. Bring to a gentle simmer.
- Mix dry ingredients together in a medium bowl. Add water and oil and stir until combined.
- Place seitan on counter top and knead like bread for about two minutes. Press seitan into a rough square shape.
- Cut into the desired number of pieces. Remember, seitan will double in size once cooked.
- Once the broth is simmering, drop seitan pieces into it. Simmer gently, uncovered, for about 30 minutes. Keep heat low so water does not actively boil.
- Remove from heat and let seitan and broth cool. Once at room temperature, transfer broth and seitan to a container. Refrigerate overnight for a firmer texture, or use immediately if desired.
- Freeze seitan in broth for later use.

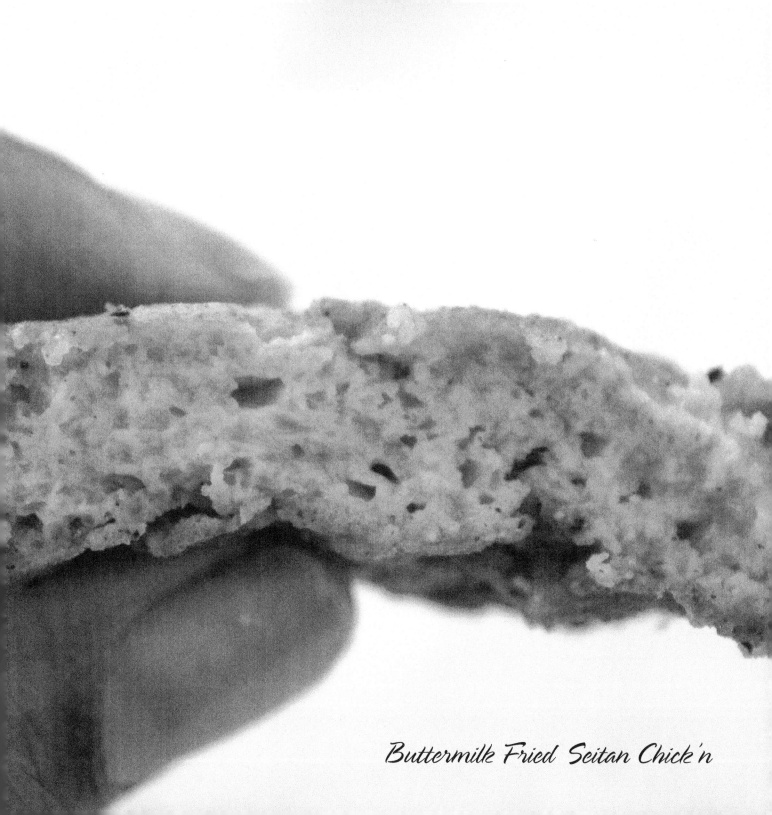

Buttermilk Fried Seitan Chick'n

Sriracha Barbecue Chick'n Sandwiches
Serves 4

I love to make these when meat eaters are coming over for a visit. The barbecue smell and taste is one they're familiar with, which makes eating a vegan meal a lot easier. Spicy Sriracha and sweet barbecue sauce blend wonderfully to create a great taste sensation. The success of this dish is dependent upon the barbecue sauce, so use a good quality one or make your own.

Ingredients

1 Tablespoon olive oil

2 shallots, minced

12 oz of previously made chick'n style seitan, cut into thin slices about an inch long

1 cup barbecue sauce

¼ cup dark beer

1 Tablespoon Sriracha (or pepper sauce of your choice)

4 burger buns, lightly toasted (or 12 slider buns)

Instructions

- Heat olive oil in large saucepan over medium heat. Add the minced shallot and sauté for 3-5 minutes, until soft.
- Add the seitan, and cook until it turns a light brown and crisp on the edges. Stir often to prevent burning.
- Add the barbecue sauce, beer and pepper sauce. Mix well. Continue cooking for another 3-5 minutes, or until sauce is thick and gooey.
- Top each burger size bun with ¼ of the seitan mix. Garnish as desired with tomato slices, lettuce, vegan coleslaw, shredded red cabbage, sliced red onions, or a sprinkle of vegan cheese.

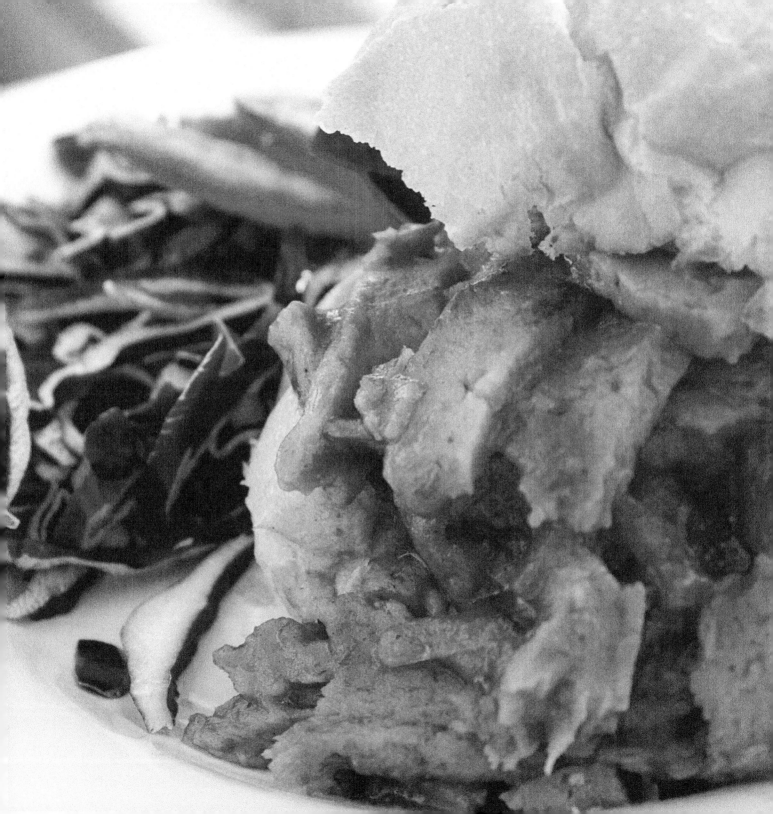

Bellylicious "Buffalo Wangz"
Serves 4

This highly rated recipe is some yummy stuff - the mouth sizzling flavor of buffalo wings without the sodium, saturated fat or calories, they're perfect for snacks, game nights or social gatherings. You can certainly use a different hot sauce, but Frank's is the traditional, the gold standard of wing sauces... and to me it tastes the best.

Ingredients

7 cups water

2 vegetable bouillon cubes

2 not-chicken bouillon cube

1 onion, quartered

3 Tablespoons garlic powder

1 Tablespoon liquid aminos

2 cups vital wheat gluten

½ cup nutritional yeast flakes

1 teaspoon seasoning salt

1 teaspoon fresh ground black pepper

1 teaspoon poultry seasoning

1 Tablespoon onion powder

1 Tablespoon garlic powder

1 cup soy milk

½ cup water

Instructions

- Combine water, broth cubes, liquid aminos, onion and garlic powder in 4 quart saucepan; bring to a simmer over medium heat.
- Combine next seven ingredients in large bowl and whisk together to mix thoroughly.
- Remove 1½ cups of broth from pot and pour into dry ingredients. Mix well with rubber spatula until all dry ingredients are incorporated, adding more broth by the Tablespoon as needed.
- Knead dough in bowl for 2 minutes, then pull small chunks off, flattening them to ½" high. Drop them into the simmering broth.
- Simmer over low heat for 45-55 minutes.
- Remove seitan "wings" from pan, drain, and place into bowl of soy milk and water; let sit for about 5 minutes to absorb the liquid.
- Remove seitan from milk a few pieces at a time, drain off excess liquid, then roll in Buffalo Wangz coating mixture.

- Place wangz on baking sheet and set aside for 1 hour.

Buffalo Wangz Coating & Sauce

1 cup cornstarch
½ cup all-purpose flour
1½ teaspoons seasoned or garlic salt
1½ teaspoons cayenne pepper
1½ teaspoons paprika
1½ teaspoons fresh ground black pepper
1 stick vegan butter, melted
1-2 teaspoons maple syrup
1 cup Frank's Red Hot sauce
peanut oil

- Mix together cornstarch, flour and spices, and coat seitan pieces thoroughly.
- Heat bit of oil in non-stick skillet, then add seitan a few pieces at a time. Fry until crisp and evenly browned.
- Remove from pan and drain on paper towels.
- Heat vegan butter over low heat. Add hot sauce and maple syrup; stir to blend. Add wings to pot and stir gently to coat with sauce. Taste and add bit of salt if desired.
- Remove, drain off excess sauce.
- Serve with celery sticks, carrot sticks and/or vegan ranch dressing.

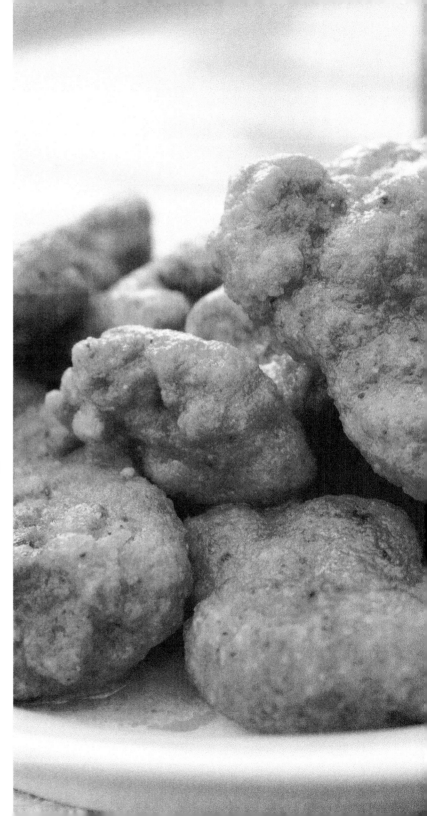

Black Bean Chili
Serves 6

My Dad's family is from Texas - the state known for cooks who make the best chili in the world. This is as good as it gets without beef. We normally eat chili over rice, or right out of the bowl with saltine crackers. Top your chili with diced red onions or pico de gallo, grated cheese, cilantro or a dollop of vegan sour cream.

Ingredients

1 lb dry black beans

1 Tablespoon olive oil

2 cups chopped white onion

1 cup chopped carrots

3 Tablespoons chili powder

1 Tablespoon minced fresh garlic

1 teaspoon ground cumin

1 teaspoon red pepper flakes

¼ teaspoon ground cinnamon

3 not-chicken or vegetable bouillon cubes

2 teaspoons oregano leaves

1 teaspoon Himalayan pink salt

Instructions

- Rinse beans and clean them by picking out any shrived, chipped or broken beans and pebbles.
- Place beans in a large bowl and add water 2" past beans.
- Heat oil in large heavy pot over medium heat. Add the onions and carrots, and cook 10 minutes stirring frequently until veggies are soft.
- Add chili powder, garlic, cumin, red pepper, and cinnamon. Cook, stirring for 1 minute. Add the beans, broth, and oregano and bring to a boil. Reduce heat and simmer, partially covered, for 90 minutes. Add salt and continue cooking another 30 minutes.
- Smash about ⅓ of the beans against the edge of the pot with the back of your cooking spoon. You want small lumps, not completely smooth bean paste. Stir until blended.
- Serve over cooked brown rice and garnish as desired.

Vegetable Stir Fry
Serves 4

Guess what I discovered? Real oyster sauce is made from oysters! (That's right up there with a question my uncle used to tease us with as kids: "who's buried in Grant's Tomb?") As there are many people allergic to shellfish who don't eat oysters just like vegans/vegetarians, vegan oyster sauce is widely available. The flavor is fabulous and no oysters will be sacrificed for your meal.

Ingredients

2 Tablespoons olive oil

2 slices of fresh ginger root, minced

1 clove garlic, minced

1½ cups broccoli florets

1 cup carrots, sliced thin

1 small onion, sliced in half and separated into rings

1 cup water, into which you dissolved

1 not-chicken broth cube

1 teaspoon sea salt

1 Tablespoon cornstarch

1 Tablespoon cold water

1 8 oz can water chestnuts, drained and sliced

1 cup sliced mushrooms

2-3 Tablespoons vegan oyster sauce (to taste)

Instructions

- Heat oil in wok or large pan over medium-high heat until hot. Add ginger root and garlic; stir-fry until light brown (about 60 seconds).
- Add broccoli, carrots and onion, stir fry another minute.
- Add the hot not-chicken broth water to the pot, along with salt. Now you cover the pan and cook until carrots are tender, but still firm (about 3 minutes).
- Mix your cornstarch and water together; add it to the vegetable mixture. Cook, stirring constantly until it thickens. This should only take 10-15 seconds.
- Toss in the water chestnuts, mushrooms and oyster sauce. Cook and stir another 30 seconds, then you're done!
- Serve over hot brown or jasmine rice.
- Add marinated tofu, sprinkle it with peanuts, or slivered almonds to up your protein content for the day.

Southern Mock Country Fried Steak and White Gravy
Serves 4-6

I'd never heard of Country (or Chicken) Fried Steak before I moved to Texas, but it became a favorite breakfast choice; however, the fat and sodium content is off the chart - plus it's made out of cow. In other words, it's a trifecta of no-no's for a vegan. For the "steak" follow the Where's the Beef-y Seitan" recipe. Breading for the patty and white gravy recipe follow.

Ingredients

-- For the Breading
1 cup unbleached flour
1 cup saltine cracker crumbs, crushed
½ teaspoon seasoning salt
½ teaspoon paprika
1 teaspoon ground black peppercorns
¼ cup vegan creamer
2 vegan eggs (flax eggs or egg replacer, prepared)

-- For the White Gravy
1 Tablespoon vegan buttermilk
3 Tablespoons olive oil
⅓ cup minced onion
⅓ cup unbleached flour
1 cup vegan creamer
1-2 cups almond milk
1 teaspoon white pepper
2 teaspoons not-chicken seasoning paste
Vegan bacon bits

Instructions

• Put ½ package (narrow strip) of crackers into a large zip style bag. Using a rolling pin, crush the crackers into medium-fine crumbs. Measure and add more as needed to make 1 cup. Dump onto a plate.
• Combine flour with black pepper, and pour into a pie plan or shallow bowl.
• Vegan eggs should be whipped well and in a shallow bowl.
• Dip each seitan steak into the egg picture, then the flour, back into the egg mixture, then into the cracker crumbs. Sit on a tray while you prepare the remaining steaks.
• Heat oil in frying pan over medium-high heat. Fry one at a time to maintain crispness of the coating (about 2 minutes) per side. You're just browning the crust, as the seitan is already cooked.
• Place on baking tray in 250 degree oven to keep warm while you finish the remainder.

-- Instructions for Making the White Gravy
- Add butter and oil to the pan; heat over medium heat until butter is melted.
- Add onion and cook until translucent. Reduce heat to low and add the flour, whisking constantly until your roux has a pale brown appearance and emits a nutty aroma. Watch it carefully because you don't want it to darken too much.
- Transfer to a bowl and mix in the creamer, milk, salt, pepper, not-chicken seasoning, and flour. Using your stick blender, whip until onion is mixed into the other ingredients.
- Transfer gravy back into pan. Add 1 Tablespoon of vegan bacon bits, salt and pepper to taste. Bring to a boil over low heat, stirring frequently until thickened.

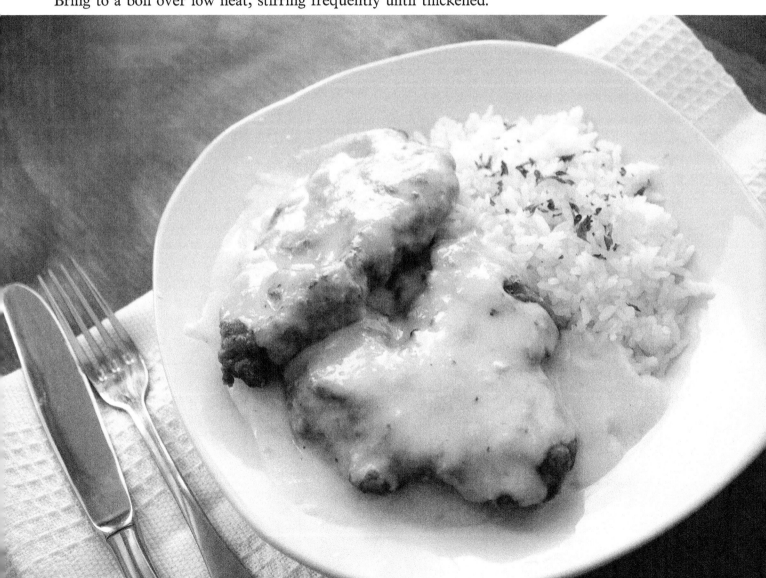

Eggplant Coconut Cream Soup
Serves 6-8

I really like eggplant; it's high in iron, and absorbs the flavors of whatever it is cooked with. Try this light, creamy soup with a salad and crusty French bread for dipping. Plain coconut creamer is good, but one day I accidentally picked up French vanilla, and was pleasantly surprised at the light but rich sweetness which gave the soup an interesting taste.

Ingredients

2 small to medium eggplants
4 cups water
1 teaspoon sea salt
2 Tablespoons vegan butter
2 Tablespoons olive oil
2 large yellow onions, finely chopped
½ cup celery, finely chopped
4 large red potatoes, peeled and sliced
1 teaspoon curry powder
¼ teaspoon cayenne
¼ teaspoon thyme leaves
½ teaspoon basil leaves
2 bay leaves
1 teaspoon Himalayan pink salt
2 not-chicken bouillon cubes
4 cups water
1 teaspoon black pepper
Few shakes of hot pepper sauce
¾ cup minced green onions, divided in half
12 oz carton coconut creamer

Instructions

- Peel and slice the eggplant and place in 4 cups water with the 1 teaspoon salt. Let eggplant slices soak for 10-15 minutes; drain, rinse and finely dice. Place in large bowl.
- Chop onions, celery and potatoes; add to bowl with diced eggplant. Add half the chopped green onions to bowl with other vegetables.
- In a small bowl combine the curry, cayenne, thyme, basil, bay leaves, and salt.
- Heat large heavy sauce pan over low heat. Add the butter and oil. When melted, add the onions, celery, potatoes and eggplant and sauté slowly for 15 minutes, stirring frequently to avoid sticking.
- Add spice mixture to pot, stir and cook 8-10 more minutes. Stir in four cups water and two not-chicken cubes, then cover pot and simmer soup for about 30 minutes, stirring occasionally.
- Remove bay leaves then puree contents of pot with immersion blender until smooth. Return to pot and add pepper sauce, remaining green onions, pepper, and coconut creamer.
- Bring to a simmer and serve.

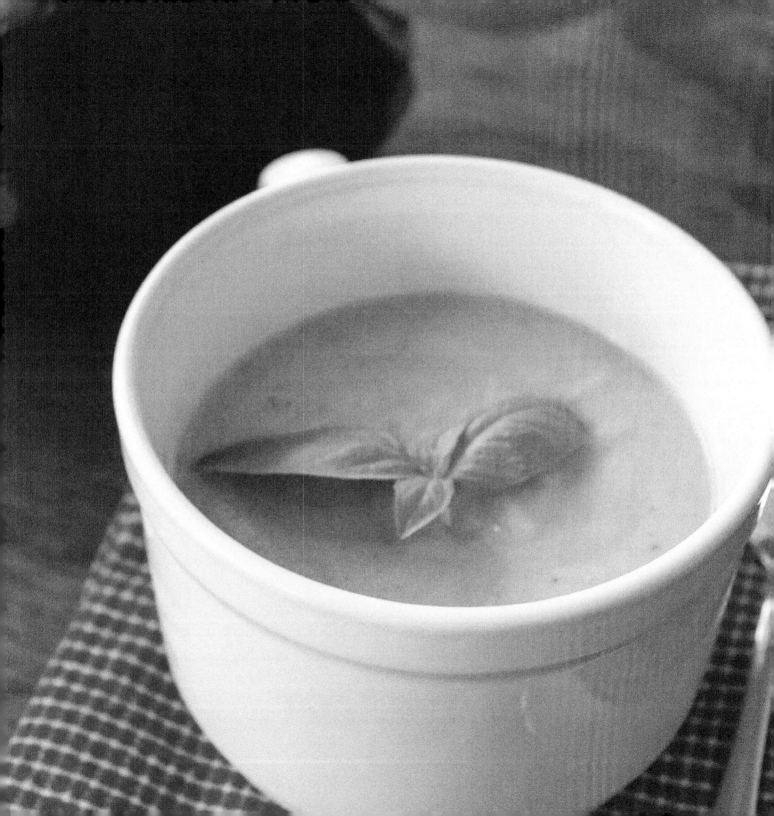

Purple and White Cole Slaw
Serves 6

A salute to my brothers and their fraternities! One wears the red and white of Kappa Alpha Psi, the other the purple and gold of Omega Psi Phi. Feel free to prepare the cabbage and carrots the day before, but wait until close to serving time to add the onions and dressing.

Ingredients

¼ medium head of both red and green cabbage, shredded fine (3 cups each)

1 large carrot, peeled and grated

2 teaspoons kosher salt (or 1 teaspoon pink salt)

½ cup vegan mayonnaise

¼ teaspoon celery seed

2 Tablespoons rice wine vinegar

Fresh ground black pepper

Instructions

• Toss the cabbage and carrots with salt in colander set over medium bowl. Let stand until cabbage wilts - at least an hour.

• Dump wilted cabbage and carrots into the bowl. Rinse thoroughly in cold water. Pour vegetables back into colander, pressing but not squeezing them to drain.

• Pat dry with paper towels. If storing to prepare later, place in zip style plastic bag and refrigerate.

• Pour cabbage and carrots back into the bowl. Add onions, mayonnaise, and vinegar. Toss to coat thoroughly.

• Season with pepper to taste. Cover and refrigerate until ready to serve.

Rice Cakes a la San Francisco
Serves 5-6

Easy to make and tasty way to use leftover rice hanging around in the fridge.

Ingredients

⅔ cup water

⅓ cup almond milk

¼ teaspoon sea salt

⅔ cup precooked rice

2 teaspoons grated onion

1 Tablespoon vegan butter

¼ cup flour

1½ teaspoons baking powder

1 teaspoon agave nectar

1 prepared vegan egg

⅛ teaspoon black pepper

Instructions

• To make a vegan egg, combine 1 Tablespoon ground flax seeds with 3 Tablespoons warm water. Whisk together and stick in the refrigerator for 1-2 minutes.

• Bring rice, salt and butter to a boil. Stir in precooked rice, then cover and remove from heat. Let stand about 5 minutes.

• Meanwhile, combine the vegan egg, almond milk, and onion, then mix with the rice.

• Mix the remaining ingredients and add them to the rice mixture, mixing only enough to dampen the flour.

• Drop by Tablespoons onto hot, greased frying pan or griddle and allow to brown lightly on both sides.

• Serve hot with jelly, syrup or jam for breakfast, or as a side dish with seitan or vegetables for dinner.

Cajun Chicken Style Seitan
Makes About 1 Pound

Cajun "chicken style" seitan can be used in a variety of dishes due to it's deep flavor and meaty texture. I've tried preparing the same recipe steamed in foil, baked, and boiled. This version gives the best results.

Ingredients

--Wet Stuff

1 cup water
1 cup vegetable broth
2 Tablespoons vegetarian chicken seasoning
2 Tablespoons olive oil
1 teaspoon Bragg's aminos
1 teaspoon vegan Worcestershire sauce

-- Dry Stuff

2 cups vital wheat gluten
⅓ cup chickpea flour
⅓ cup nutritional yeast flakes
½ teaspoon black pepper
1½ teaspoons baking powder
1 Tablespoon garlic powder
2 teaspoons poultry seasoning
¾ teaspoon sweet paprika
¼ teaspoon white pepper
½ teaspoon cayenne pepper
2 teaspoons Cajun style seasoning of choice

Instructions

- In a small bowl, mix together wet ingredients with fork or whisk until blended; set aside.
- Place all dry ingredients in a large bowl and whisk together until well blended. Create a hole in the center and slowly pour the wet ingredients into it, mixing with a rubber spatula. Scrape sides of bowl to mix in flours and seasonings.
- Transfer dough to counter and knead it for 3 minutes. Really dig in there to develop the sticky gluten, which will hold the seitan together.
- Return seitan to bowl and let dough sit for about 20 minutes to rest.
- Remove from bowl and knead another 30 seconds as you try to pull and shape the dough into a 2" thick square.

- Cut seitan so you end up with 8-16 pieces (depending on recipe you're making). Be sure to flatten and stretch the pieces to about 1" thickness.

Make the Simmering Broth
- Place 3 cups of water, 3 cups of low sodium vegetable stock, two Tablespoons tamari sauce or Bragg's Aminos, and one Tablespoon Cajun style seasoning in large pot.
- Drop in pieces of flattened seitan dough. Cover pot and heat to boil, then reduce to barely a simmer.
- Cook for 50-60 minutes, then remove from heat.
- Let cool in pot, then remove and place on rack to drain.

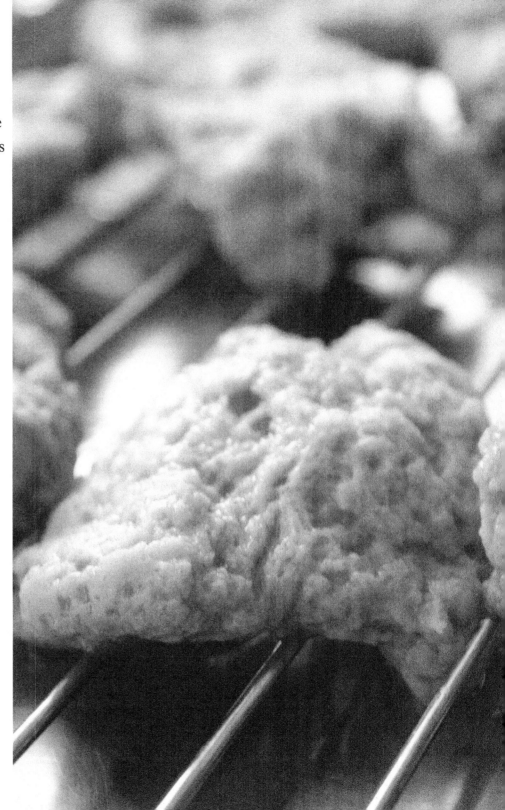

Roasted Vegetables
Makes 6 Cups

Have you ever tried roasting vegetables? It's super easy and a great way to up your intake of vegetables almost effortlessly. Great eating with meals or as snacks. Even children enjoy snacking on roasted vegetables, and they're great to have as an energy booster at the office to prevent forays to the candy or chip machine. Parsnips, sweet potatoes, red onion, cauliflower, beets, green beans, and okra are all excellent vegetables to try roasting as well.

Ingredients

2 carrots scrubbed and cut in half lengthwise, then into 1" pieces

1 head broccoli, cut into 2" florets

1 pound small Brussels sprouts, cut in half

2 red potato, cut into 1" chunks

½ pound green beans, cut into 2" pieces

Instructions

- Preheat oven to 400 degrees.
- Toss vegetables in a large bowl with sea salt, black pepper and olive oil until well seasoned and covered lightly in oil.
- Place in roasting pan or shallow baking tray and roast in oven until browned on the edges.
- Be sure to flip vegetables so both sides can be done evenly.

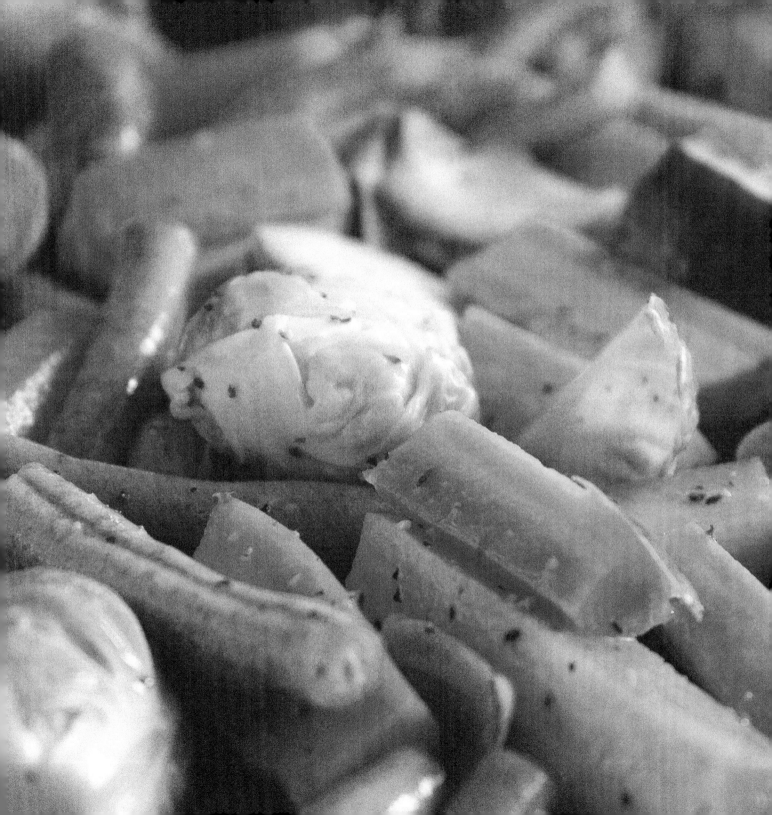

California Black Bean Burgers with Secret Sauce
Serves 4-6

Living in California provides the opportunity to try dozens of different types of peppers grown within the state. I call this burger the "California Black Bean Burger" because it makes use of Anaheim peppers, which are native to Southern California. This deep green, 5-6" long, mildly hot pepper offers a rich, but mellow flavor. If you can't find Anaheim peppers in your area, substitute Poblano or green bell peppers.

Ingredients

1 15 oz can of organic black beans, rinsed and drained

3 Tablespoons water

1 teaspoon vegan egg replacer mixed in ¼ cup water

½ red onion, cut into 4 pieces

1 Anaheim chile, seeded and cut into chunks

3 large cloves garlic, peeled

1 Tablespoon chili powder

1 teaspoon dried onion flakes

1 teaspoon seasoned salt

1 teaspoon ground cumin

½ teaspoon fresh ground black pepper

1 teaspoon Sriracha hot sauce

¾ cup rolled oats

Instructions

- Mix egg replacement with water per instructions and set aside. Rinse and drain black beans and set aside.
- Measure out cumin, chili powder, dried onion flakes and Sriracha, then add to egg replacer mixture.
- Put onion chunks in food processor and pulse a few times. Add peppers and garlic, pulse a lil' bit more. Add oats and pulse 6-8 times to blend. Add egg replacer/spice mixture and beans, then pulse until lumpy paste forms.
- Spray a sheet of aluminum foil thoroughly with non-stick spray and lay it over a baking sheet.
- Divide the bean mixture into 6 patties, forming them about ¼" thick. (The circumference of the patties should

116

correspond to the buns you're using; smaller buns = more patties).

- Stick patties and baking sheet in freezer for about 30 minutes.
- If you plan to bake your burgers, preheat oven to 375 degrees and bake for 15 minutes per side.
- If you prefer to grill your patties, trim foil around each frozen patty and put it, foil and all, on a hot grill. Cook 7-9 minutes per side.
- If you like pan-fried burgers better, place a small amount of oil in a non-stick frying pan and heat over medium, frying frozen patty until brown and crispy (about 6-7 minutes per side).
- Pan frying the baked burgers is a great way to crisp them up and make sure they are firm instead of mushy in the middle. A Foreman style grill works well too.
- Secret Sauce recipe in Sauces & Dressings section (page 28).

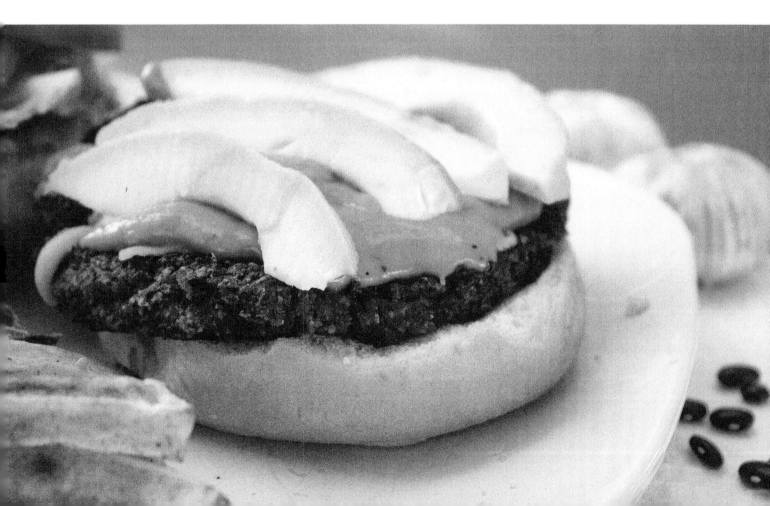

Chickpea "Meatballs"
Makes About 20

Continuing the trend of finding some way to use the tons of fresh basil available around here, combined with my favorites (chickpeas), these little balls of flavor are light in texture, but firm and delicious. They aren't meant to be simmered in sauce, but do hold up well when covered with pasta sauce or gravy right before serving.

Ingredients

2 cups cooked chickpeas, drained of water

1½ cups oat flour (ground oats)

1 cup rolled oats

2 Tablespoons ground flax seeds

¼ teaspoon red pepper flakes

½ teaspoon Himalayan pink salt

2 Tablespoons nutritional yeast flakes

½ teaspoon smoked paprika

¼ cup chopped fresh basil leaves

½ not-chicken broth cube dissolved in

1 cup warm water

1 teaspoon crushed dried oregano leaves

1 heaping teaspoon garlic powder

1 heaping teaspoon onion powder

Panko bread crumbs

Peanut oil

Instructions

- Mix ingredients together and let sit for 30-45 minutes on counter.
- Pour about 1 cup of panko bread crumbs into shallow bowl.
- Using about 1 Tablespoon of batter, form small balls.
- Roll ball in panko bread crumbs and place on plate.
- Heat 2 cups peanut or other oil to frying temperature in small saucepan.
- Deep fry chickpea meatballs a few at a time until toasty brown.
- Remove from oil and drain on paper towel.

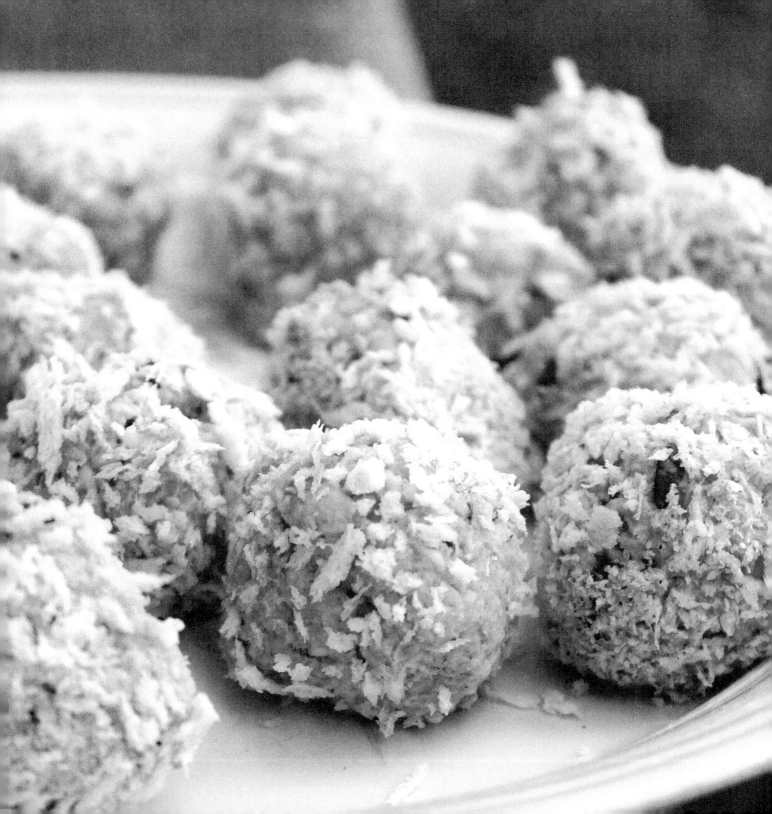

Black Bean, Rice & Cheeze Baked Burritos
Serves 8-10

With a double batch of Spicy Black Beans in the fridge, and my cousin and her children coming for a visit, I whipped up a batch of these at the last minute, created from things I scrounged up. Surprise! They went over really well. The kids gave them a solid 9.5 on a scale of 1-10.

Ingredients

2 cups Spicy Black Beans or Cuban Black Beans

1 cup leftover rice

1 8 oz carton pico de gallo salsa

1 package vegan cheeze shreds (cheddar or Mexican style)

8-10 artisan burrito wraps

Instructions

• Preheat oven to 400 degrees.

• Spray 13x9" baking dish with non-stick baking spray.

• Place beans, rice, ⅔ of cheeze and salsa in large bowl and mix thoroughly.

• Spoon about ⅔ cup of filling mixture onto ⅓ of the burrito wrap. Fold sides in, then roll tortilla up. Place seam side down in baking pan.

• Repeat until pan is full. Sprinkle burritos with remaining cheeze shreds.

• Cover pan with aluminum foil and bake for 20 minutes.

• Let sit about 5 minutes before removing from pan to firm up.

• Serve with toppings such as avocado slices, guacamole, vegan sour cream, salsa, shredded lettuce, chopped onion, sliced olives, cilantro, or additional pico de gallo.

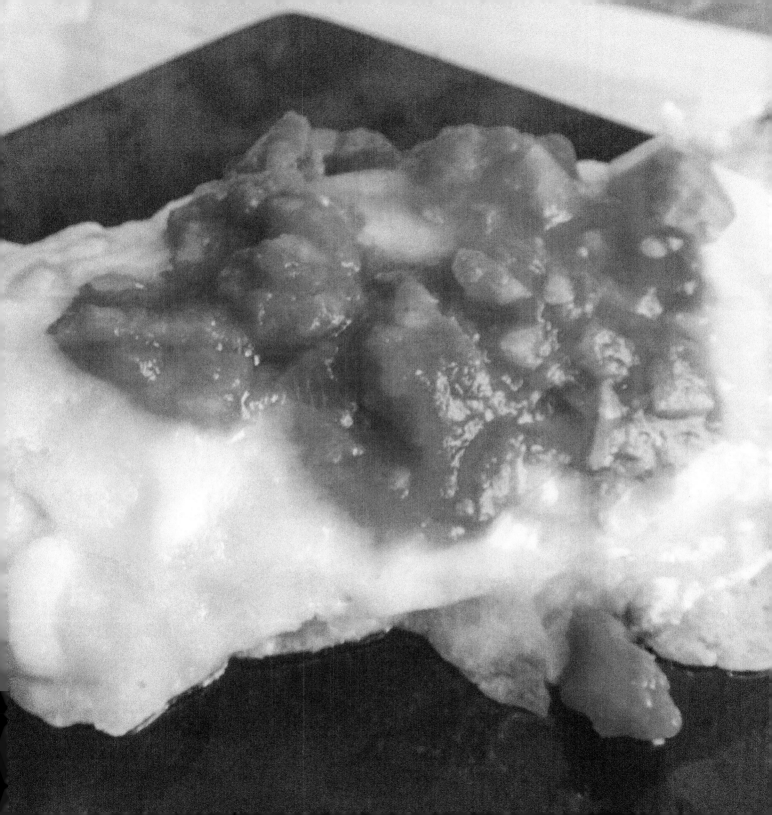

Vegetable Pizza on the Grill
Makes 1 Medium Pizza

The weather in the San Francisco Bay Area is pretty mild, so we grill a lot. I'm so bad I will stand out in the rain with my umbrella in one hand and my tongs in the other. This pizza provides the smoky flavor of hickory or mesquite in the vegetables, so it tastes like pizzeria pizza. Use a premade crust and commercial vegan mozzarella to speed up mealtime preparation.

Ingredients

1 medium prepared pizza crust

1 red bell pepper, cut into quarters with seeds removed

1 small zucchini, sliced

1 small eggplant, sliced

6 large ripe tomatoes, halved with seeds removed

2 Tablespoons pesto sauce

Salt and fresh ground black pepper to taste

1 heaping cup (5-6 oz) shredded vegan mozzarella cheese shreds

Instructions

• Preheat oven to 450 degrees.

• Place pizza stone or baking sheet on the top shelf to preheat.

• Brush bell peppers, zucchini, eggplant and onion with a little olive oil, and place on the grill over hot coals until charred all over.

• Place tomato halves (skin side up) on the grill rack and cook until blisters form. Peel off and discard skin.

• Mash roasted tomato with pesto sauce, salt and pepper.

• Spread tomato mixture over pizza crust, and arrange grilled vegetables over the top.

• Sprinkle mozzarella over vegetables and transfer to hot pizza stone/baking sheet.

• Bake for 25-30 minutes or until cheese turns golden brown and sauce is bubbling.

Tempeh Mock Chicken Salad
Makes 1½ Cups

I've taken this to many different potlucks over the years, and it was always well received. Great on sandwiches, as a salad topper, or with crackers as a snack.

Ingredients

1 8 oz package of tempeh

4 Tablespoons vegan mayonnaise

1 Tablespoon nutritional yeast

1 Tablespoon gherkin pickles, chopped fine

2 Tablespoons minced fresh parsley

1 teaspoon Dijon mustard

1 teaspoon tamari

1 large stalk celery, diced

¼ medium onion, diced

Instructions

• Place tempeh in steamer basket, cover and steam for 15 minutes. Remove from heat, let cool, and dice into ¼" squares.

• Combine tempeh with the remaining ingredients and mix well.

• Refrigerate for an hour or more before serving to allow tempeh to absorb the flavors.

• Store in the refrigerator.

Grilled Vegetable Shish Kabobs
Serves 4

As a child I wanted to "shish kabob" everything. I thought it was so cool to walk around eating dinner off a stick. Which it really is. Veggie kabobs are a great side dish for grilled bean burgers, grilled tofu, or pasta.

Ingredients

1 large eggplant, cut into bite-sized pieces
½ large red bell pepper, seeded and cut into 1" squares
½ large yellow bell pepper, seeded and cut into 1" squares
2 zucchini, trimmed and cut into ½" slices
2 yellow squash, trimmed and cut into ½" slices
8 shallots, quartered
16 small cremini or button mushrooms
16 cherry tomatoes
Fresh oregano and parsley sprigs (for garnish)
--Marinade
½ cup olive oil
1 Tablespoon raspberry vinegar
½ teaspoon sea salt
½ teaspoon fresh ground black pepper
1 teaspoon dry mustard
1 Tablespoon light brown sugar
1 clove garlic, minced
1 Tablespoon chopped fresh oregano
1 Tablespoon chopped fresh parsley

Instructions

• Mix together the olive oil, raspberry vinegar, salt, pepper, mustard, brown sugar, oregano, garlic and parsley. Stir until well blended.

• Place eggplant in a colander and sprinkle with salt. Cover with a plate to weigh it down and leave it for 30 minutes (this extracts the excess water). Rinse eggplant under running tap to remove salt, then press out any water it has absorbed.

• Add vegetables to marinade, turning to coat them evenly. Cover with plastic wrap and let marinate for about an hour.

• Thread mixture of vegetables onto skewers, alternating so there are a variety of tastes on each one.

• Cook over hot coals 3-5 minutes until tender-crisp, brushing with marinade as you turn kabobs to cook on all sides.

• Arrange on serving platter, then garnish with fresh oregano and parsley.

Chickpea & Okra Stir Fry
Serves 4-6

Okra is a starring vegetable in restaurants and on home menus all through the southern United States, and with good reason. Okra is a nutritional powerhouse, providing a rich source of Vitamins A, B, and C, folic acid, potassium, and fiber.

Ingredients

1 lb okra, ends trimmed

2 Tablespoons olive oil

1 Tablespoon vegan butter

1 large yellow onion, chopped fine

1 clove garlic, minced

3 Roma tomatoes, chopped

1 Serrano or jalapeño pepper, white pith and seeds removed

1 teaspoon grated fresh ginger

1 Tablespoon cumin

1 Tablespoon cilantro, chopped

1 can organic chickpeas (garbanzo beans), drained and rinsed

Salt and pepper to taste

Instructions

• Using a wok or large frying pan, heat oil and vegan butter.

• Sauté the onion and garlic for a few minutes, until the onion is soft.

• Add tomatoes, green chile, and ginger; stir well. Then add the okra, cumin and coriander.

• Cover pan and cook over medium-high heat, stirring frequently (stir frying) to prevent sticking, for about 2 minutes.

• Add chickpeas, salt and pepper.

• Continue cooking until chickpeas are heated through.

• Serve over fluffy jasmine, brown or basmati rice

Perfectly Fluffy Rice Every Time
Makes 3 Cups

More people burn, under cook, flood their stoves, and make mush out of their rice! I learned this technique from my uncle, but discovered the hard way that the techniques are slightly different for white vs. brown rice. Either way, the end result is firm textured, fluffy rice you'll be proud to serve. Results tend to be unreliable cooking less than one cup of rice, so I don't recommend it. Start with 1 cup of rice and a heavy bottomed saucepan with a tight-fitting lid.

Ingredients

2 teaspoons vegan butter or olive oil

1 cup long grain white or Jasmine rice

1½ cups water

½ teaspoon salt

Instructions

- Start by heating the vegan butter or olive oil over medium heat. Use a pan that is large enough for the amount of rice you'll have once it absorbs water (rice expands to 3x its original amount).
- Add rice and cook, stirring constantly, for 2-3 minutes. The goal here is to lightly toast the rice, developing a nice nutty flavor.
- Add the water all at once, along with the salt. Stir once. Bring mixture to a boil.
- Immediately reduce heat to low, cover the pot tightly, and simmer until liquid is absorbed (about 15 minutes). Do not remove the top to peek!
- Turn off the burner, and let rice sit for another 12-15 minutes as it slowly finishes cooking and absorbing the steam.
- If you use basmati rice, it will be ready at the 15 minute mark without the additional steaming.

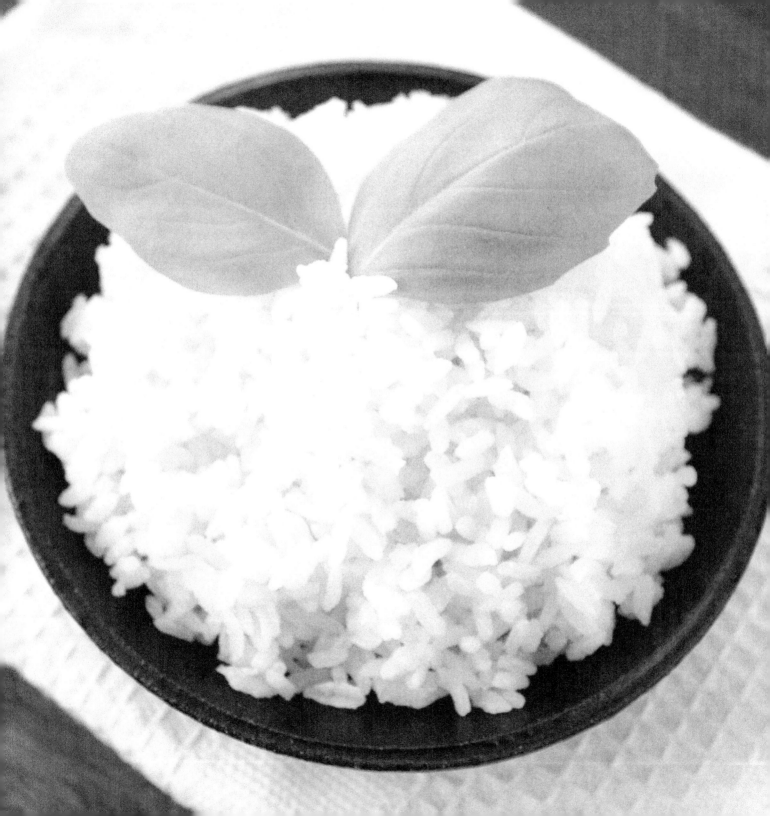

Technique for Perfect Brown Rice
Serves 4

Suitable for either long or short grain brown rice, wild rice, and even black rice.

Ingredients

6 cups water

1 cup brown rice

2 teaspoons olive oil or vegan butter

1 teaspoon sea salt

Instructions

- Bring water to a boil in a medium-sized pot. Stir in rice, oil/butter, and salt. With water at a brisk simmer, cook the rice, uncovered, until it's almost tender (about 30 minutes).
- Drain rice into a steamer basket that fits inside the pot. Fill pot with about 1" of water, and return it to the stove.
- Place basket of rice inside pot, cover and steam over low heat until tender, about 8-10 minutes.
- Scoop rice into a bowl and fluff gently with a fork before serving to separate the grains.

Cashew-Based Cheeze Sauce
Makes 1½ Cups

This sauce serves as the foundation for many vegan dishes which call for cheese, such as macaroni and cheeze, quesadillas, nachos, cheeze sandwiches, pizza topping, dip and more.

Ingredients

2 cups raw cashews, soaked at least 3 hours and drained

1 cup water

¾ cup nutritional yeast flakes

½ teaspoon granulated onion

¼ teaspoon white pepper

¼ teaspoon sea salt

Instructions

- Blend all ingredients together in high speed blender until smooth.
- Refrigerate immediately in container with air-tight lid.
- Use within 7-10 days.

Grilled Cheeze Sandwiches with Tomato & Basil
Serves 4

I love basil, evidenced by the fact that we have four basil plants on my patio. These open-faced cheeze sandwiches are a tasty snack or light lunch that puts my beloved basil together with two of my favorite things - fresh organic tomatoes and cashew cheeze. A toaster oven gives best results. Watch closely or you'll have overly toasted bread like I did. Yet, surprisingly, no one complained and they disappeared within seconds...

Ingredients

3 Tablespoons olive oil

4 Roma tomatoes, chopped fine

20 leaves fresh basil, torn into small pieces (use more or less to taste)

½ teaspoon Kosher salt (or to taste)

½ teaspoon fresh ground black pepper (or to taste)

6 ¾" slices of Italian, French, sourdough or other heavy crusted bread

1 clove garlic, peeled and cut in half lengthwise

½ cup cheeze sauce (page 129) or commercial vegan mozzarella

Instructions

• Heat olive oil in a small sauté pan. Add tomatoes and basil, and season with the salt and pepper to taste. Cook over to low to medium heat for about 8 minutes, or until the tomato juices are gone.

• Lightly toast the bread. When it has cooled slightly but is still hot, rub it on one side with the garlic slices.

• Spread a bit of the tomato mix on each piece of bread with the back of a spoon, then top it with the cheeze or vegan mozzarella.

• Place on baking sheet and place under broiler in oven. When cheeze begins to turn slightly brown and bread is toasted (only takes about 2 minutes), remove from oven.

• Best served hot.

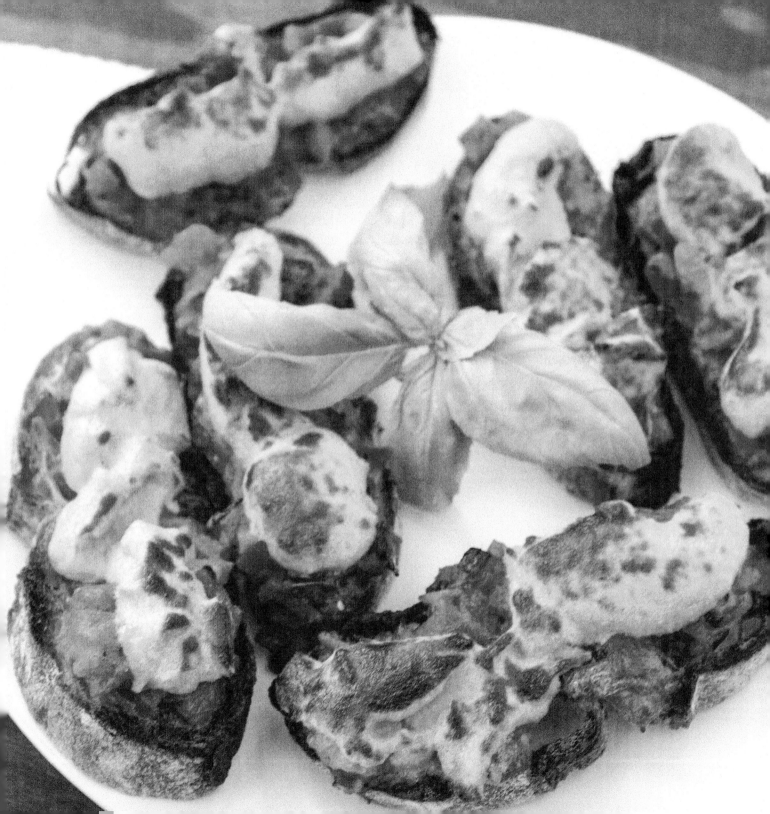

Thai Basil Fried Rice with Seitan
Serves 3-4

Try this fabulous version of spicy Thai basil fried rice which uses chicken-style seitan in place of ground chicken, and vegan oyster sauce in place of the shellfish-based version. Purchase Thai basil, chile peppers, long beans, vegan fish sauce, and vegan oyster sauce at an Asian market.

Ingredients

4 cloves of garlic, minced

1 red and 1 green Thai chile pepper, sliced fine

½ cup chicken style seitan, cut into ¼" chunks

⅓ cup onion, sliced and cut into 1" pieces

½ cup Chinese long beans, cut into 1" pieces

⅓ cup red and green bell pepper, cut into narrow strips, then into ½" pieces

¼ cup baby carrots, cut into quarters lengthwise, then into small pieces

⅔ cup Thai basil leaves, sliced

1 Tablespoon vegan oyster sauce

2 teaspoons vegan fish sauce

1½ teaspoons double black thick soy sauce

2 teaspoons tamari

2½ cups previously cooked basmati or jasmine rice, cooled or cold from refrigerator

2 Tablespoons peanut oil

Instructions

• Prepare the ingredients, readying them in individual containers. Put the sauces in one container.

• Heat 2 Tablespoons oil in large heavy non-stick skillet over medium heat until hot. Add garlic and chopped chilies, and stir fry rapidly until garlic begins to turn brown. Make sure you do not burn it.

• Add the chopped seitan and stir fry about 60 seconds. Add the long beans, carrots and bell peppers. Stir to mix. Add in the four blended sauces.

• Continue stir frying another minute or two, then add the onion and stir fry until they are slightly limp.

• Make sure there are no clumps in your rice, then add it to the sauce mix. Flip around with a spatula to mix everything together. Add the basil and remove pan from heat. Flip mixture 5-6 more times then serve.

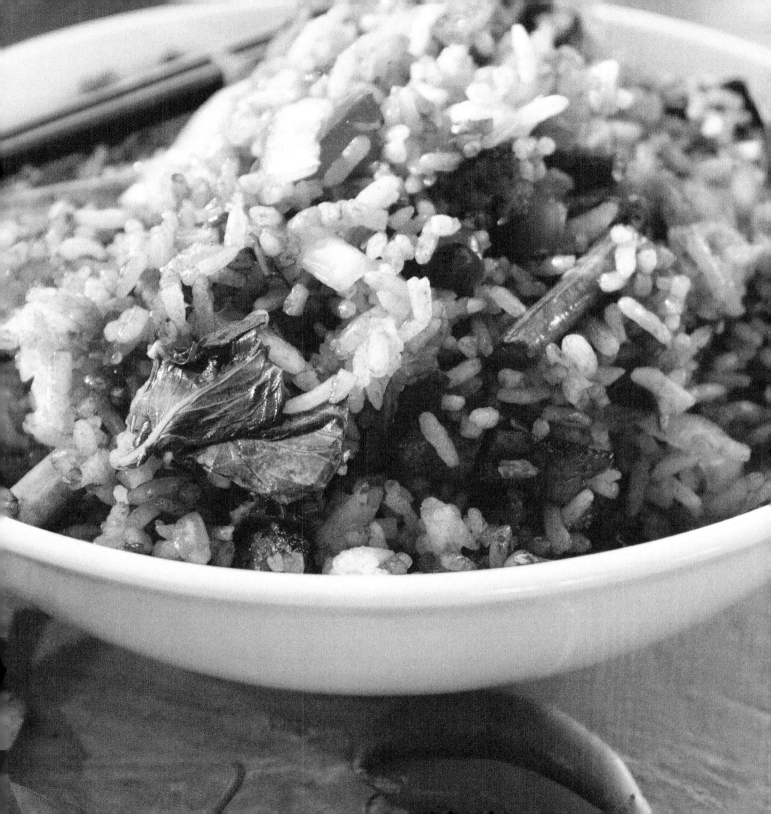

Garlic Mashed Potatoes
Makes 4-6 Servings

This recipe was inspired by Alton Brown over at The Food Network. I love garlic mashed potatoes, and tried his recipe about eight years ago when I still cooked with dairy products. Once I went vegan, I was wracking my brain to figure out how to keep the rich, creamy texture and garlicky flavor while ditching the milk and cheese. Here's what I came up with. These potatoes go really well with vegan fried chick'n and greens.

Ingredients

2 pounds russet potatoes

1 Tablespoon kosher salt

¾ cup plain soy creamer

2 large cloves garlic, minced

2 Tablespoons vegan butter

4 oz vegan Parmesan cheeze

1-2 Tablespoons chopped parsley

Fresh ground black pepper

Instructions

- Peel the potatoes and cut into chunks about 2" in size. Try to make the pieces as uniform as possible so they cook evenly.
- Add to pot with kosher salt and enough water to cover potatoes. Bring to boil over medium heat and cook until potatoes are tender. Drain potatoes into large bowl.
- In a small saucepan, warm the soy creamer, vegan butter and garlic until it begins to simmer. Pour mixture into potatoes. Add vegan Parmesan and mash with ricer (or use electric mixer), to combine until light and fluffy.
- Stir in parsley, adding more salt and pepper as needed.
- Let mix sit for a few minutes to thicken before serving.

Buttermilk Fried Chick'n Seitan
Serves 6

New vegans usually have fresh memories of juicy buttermilk fried chicken. Seitan can be seasoned so well that you'll never miss eating fried chicken. The same delicious crunch, the same juicy flavors in your mouth, and an amazingly similar texture are a delightful surprise. This recipe will help make the transition to vegan eating much smoother for those who struggle with giving up a soul and fast-food favorite.

Ingredients

1 recipe seasoned flour mix for fried chick'n (page 136)
1 cup soy creamer or almond milk
1 teaspoon apple cider vinegar or fresh lemon juice
Cooking oil

Instructions

- Pour soy or almond milk into large non-metallic cup; add 1 teaspoon vinegar or lemon juice and stir. Let sit for about 10 minutes to curdle and create "buttermilk."
- Quickly dip seitan pieces in "buttermilk," then in seasoned flour. Place on a tray in a single layer.
- Repeat this step until all pieces of seitan are coated.
- Chill in refrigerator for about an hour so that coating will adhere to chick'n.
- Fry in cooking oil until golden brown, about 2-3 minutes per side (depending upon thickness of seitan pieces).

Seasoned Flour Mix for Fried Chick'n
Makes 1¼ Cups

Use this with your favorite commercial seitan, or one made from this book.

Ingredients

1 cup unbleached all purpose flour

1 Tablespoon arrowroot powder

2 teaspoons garlic powder

1 teaspoon paprika

1 teaspoon ground black pepper

2 teaspoons seasoning salt

1 teaspoon granulated onion

¼ teaspoon dry mustard

½ teaspoon poultry seasoning

¼ teaspoon cayenne pepper

Instructions

• Place all ingredients in a gallon size plastic zip style bag. Shake to mix well.

• Using boiled chick'n style seitan, dip seitan pieces in "buttermilk," then roll in seasoning mix. Refrigerate as instructed.

• Fry over medium heat in hot oil, turning when browned.

Sautéed Kale with Garlic & Pepper
Serves 4-5

The traditional southern method of cooking greens I learned from my grandmother involved boiling them half to death in water that had been seasoned with salt pork. My mom refused to use salt pork in anything, and instead used smoked ham shanks and added Serrano peppers. One of my aunts married a Muslim and gave up pork altogether so she started seasoning her greens with smoked turkey, adding red pepper flakes at the end. All of the methods produced delicious greens, but going vegan meant trying to find a way to preserve the flavor without animal fat or smoked meat. This recipe delivers great flavor that is a combination of what I learned from female family members. Hope you like it as much as I do.

Ingredients

2 bunches kale, large stems removed and leaves cut in ½" strips

2 Tablespoons olive oil

3 cloves garlic, minced

1½ cups hot water

1 Tablespoon not-chicken seasoning paste

½ teaspoon crushed red pepper flakes

1 Serrano pepper, thinly sliced

½ teaspoon Himalayan pink salt (or to taste)

¼ teaspoon fresh ground black pepper

2-3 Tablespoons balsamic vinegar

Instructions

• Place olive oil and minced garlic in a large pot. Over medium heat, cook garlic in oil until soft and fragrant, but not browned (it will turn bitter if overcooked).

• Add the water, seasoning paste, sliced kale, Serrano pepper and red pepper flakes to pot and stir well. Cover and cook 5-8 minutes, stirring every few minutes.

• Remove cover, stir, and continue to cook until liquid has almost completely evaporated.

• Season with salt, black pepper and vinegar to taste. Pepper sauce or flakes at the table with additional vinegar works well.

Corn, Okra and Tomato Gumbo
Serves 6-8

Everyone in the South eats okra, which is where I first became acquainted with it. Cooked correctly, it has none of the sliminess that is used as the excuse to avoid this fabulous vegetable, rich in antioxidants. This gumbo is best in the summer months when corn, okra and tomatoes are fresh and in season, though frozen organic corn or okra can be easily substituted.

Ingredients

6 ears of fresh corn

2 cups cut-up okra

⅓ cup vegan butter

2 Tablespoons Magic Vegan Bacon Grease

3 medium tomatoes, chopped rough

1 Tablespoon sugar

1½ teaspoons seasoning salt

½ teaspoon black pepper

Instructions

- Shave the corn from the cobs into a large bowl. You should end up with about 4 cups of corn.
- Melt butter in large frying pan over medium heat, and cook okra until tender (about 6-7 minutes).
- Add corn and vegan bacon grease; cook, uncovered about 10 minutes.
- Stir in the remaining ingredients and continue cooking uncovered until the tomatoes are heated through (3-5 minutes).
- Serve over fluffy hot rice.

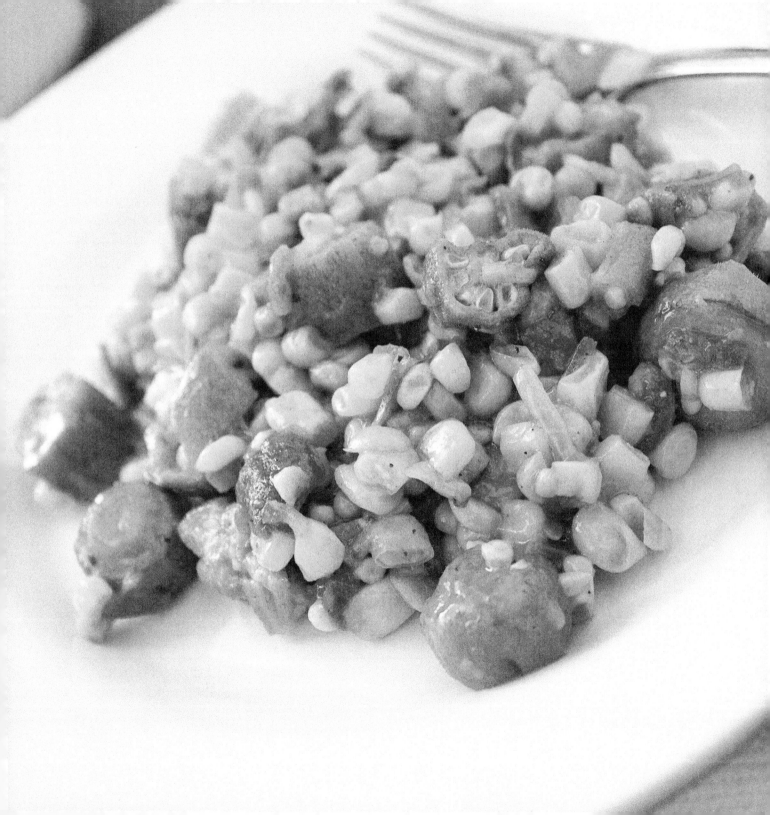

Egyptian Style Falafel
Makes 30

Falafel, hummus, tabbouleh, and baba ghanoush are some of my favorite foods. I love anything made out of chickpeas, and falafel in pita topped with tahini sauce has been lunch hundreds of times. To me, the best falafel (fluffy in texture with a delicious flavor), is made by soaking but not cooking the chickpeas.

Ingredients

2 cups dried chickpeas (cleaned)
1 cup onion, chopped
¼ cup fresh parsley, chopped
1 teaspoon baking soda
4 cloves garlic
2 Tablespoons chickpea flour
2 teaspoons salt
2 teaspoons cumin
1 teaspoon ground coriander
¼ teaspoon fresh ground black pepper
⅛ teaspoon ground cardamom

Instructions

- Wash and clean chickpeas, removing any broken or disfigured ones.
- Place cleaned chickpeas in large glass or plastic bowl and cover with cold water. Soak at least 24 hours.
- Rinse and drain soaked chickpeas, then place in food processor. Add onion, garlic, chickpea flour, baking soda, salt, cumin, coriander, pepper, parsley, and cardamom.
- Pulse repeatedly, scraping the sides of food processor regularly, until a rough coarse meal forms, then pulse a few more times. Mixture should be rough textured, not pasty and smooth like hummus or peanut butter.
- Remove into large bowl and stir, removing any chickpeas that remain whole. Cover bowl with plastic wrap and refrigerate for several hours.
- Add 2" of oil to small frying pan and heat over medium. Dampen hands and shape 1-2 Tablespoons of mix into small, slightly flattened balls.
- Drop into hot oil and brown about 3 minutes per side.
- Drain on paper towel, then serve with hummus and vegan tahini sauce, or over a salad.

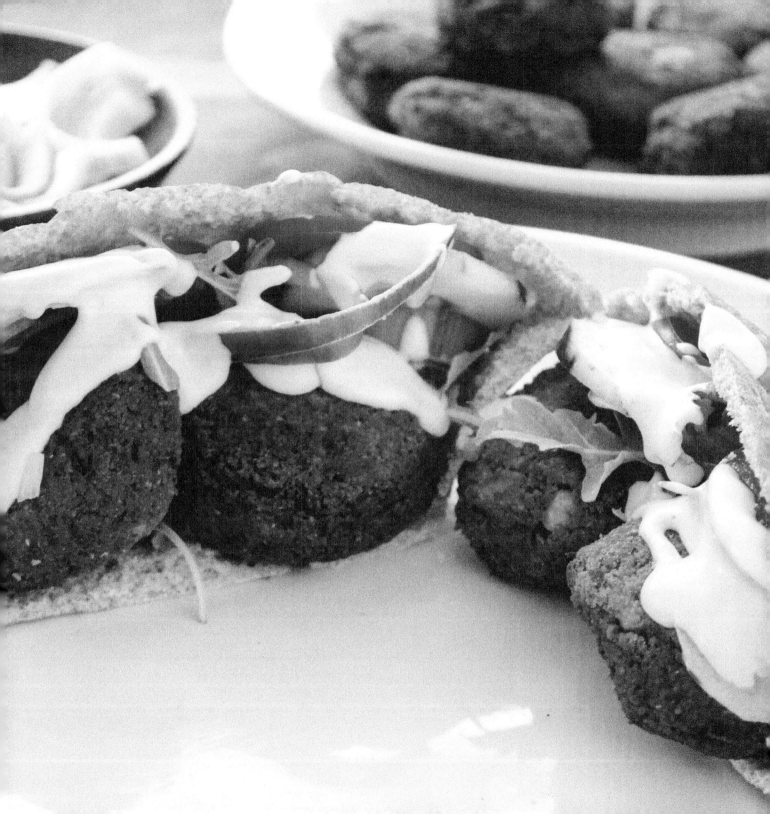

Vegan Tahini Sauce
Makes 8 oz

If you're unfamiliar with Meyer lemons, you should make your acquaintance soon. These canary yellow lemons are thinner skinned, less acidic, and quite a bit sweeter than regular lemons. You'll know immediately that something is different when you cut one open and are met with the aroma of oranges, honey and lemon.

Ingredients

1 6 oz carton of soy or almond plain non-dairy yogurt

¼ cup sesame tahini

1 large clove fresh garlic

1 teaspoon kosher salt

¼ teaspoon fresh ground black pepper

1 large Meyer lemon, juiced

Instructions

• Blend all ingredients in blender or food processor until smooth (I use a stick blender and tall narrow container for this).

• If sauce is too thick, add more lemon juice or a Tablespoon or two of water or almond milk until sauce reaches desired consistency.

• Drizzle on falafel in pita, or use as a salad dressing.

Crispy Crunchy Baked Tofu
Serves 4

Not everyone can eat soy, and certainly not everyone likes tofu. However, if you enjoy tofu as much as I do, crunchy tofu topped with your favorite sauce is a fabulous high protein snack treat. You can also put this stuff between bread with lettuce and tomato, and make it a sandwich filling.

Ingredients

1 pound of firm or extra firm water-packed tofu, drained and pressed

1 Tablespoon nutritional yeast flakes

½ teaspoon onion powder

½ teaspoon garlic powder

1 cup panko bread crumbs

¼ teaspoon seasoned or plain salt

¼ cup olive oil

Instructions

- Preheat oven to 350 degrees.
- Cut tofu into 12 slices, about ¼" thick, and place on plate.
- Combine bread crumbs, nutritional yeast, onion and garlic powders, and salt. Mix well.
- Spread 2 Tablespoons olive oil over baking sheet.
- Pour balance of olive oil over tofu and rub it around with your hands to make sure all pieces are evenly coated.
- Take one slice, coat it with the seasoned breadcrumb mixture, then place it on the oiled baking sheet. Repeat until all pieces have been coated.
- Bake for about 15 minutes, then turn over. Continue baking until tofu is light golden brown and crispy.
- Serve with Secret Sauce, barbecue sauce, ketchup or hot pepper sauce or just plain.

Spicy Black Bean & Tofu Tacos
Serves 6

These tacos are so good! Served on whole wheat or artisan tortillas, they were absolutely delicious and given a "10" by the omni and vegetarian tasting crew. Believe me, no one in your family will be thinking about meat as they stuff their faces with these puppies .

Ingredients

1 16 oz pack of extra firm dry packed tofu
2 teaspoons Ancho chili powder
½ heaping teaspoon dried oregano
½ heaping teaspoon ground cumin
½ heaping teaspoon ground coriander
½ teaspoon Himalayan pink salt
⅓ cup not-chicken or vegetable broth
1 Tablespoon olive oil
1 teaspoon onion powder
3 cloves garlic, minced
4 green onions, finely chopped
1 15 oz. can black beans, drained and rinsed
12 tortillas (warmed)
3 cups shredded romaine lettuce
1 cup pico de gallo (and more for topping)
1½ cups vegan Mexican style or cheddar cheeze strips
1 container vegan sour cream topping
Mexican hot sauce

Instructions

• Put tofu, chili powder, oregano, cumin, coriander, onion powder, and salt into a bowl and mash together thoroughly with a fork.
• Heat oil in a large non-stick skillet over medium heat. Add garlic and two-thirds of the green onions. Cook until fragrant, about 2 minutes.
• Add tofu mix and broth, and continue cooking, stirring occasionally, until most of the moisture has evaporated (10 minutes).
• Add drained beans and remaining green onions to pan. Stir well and heat until beans are warmed through, another 2-3 minutes.
• Spoon a couple of Tablespoons into tortillas, then top with lettuce, pico de gallo, cheeze strips, and a dollop of sour cream topping.
• Add a few shakes of hot sauce if you can handle the heat.

Big Ole Pot of Smoky Mixed Greens
Serves 6

My family never cooked just ONE type of greens - there was always a mixture in the pot of collards, mustards (sometimes Chinese mustards), kale and turnip greens. Seasoned of course, with salt pork, bacon or a leftover ham bone. That was then, this is now.

Ingredients

10 cups of mixed greens (about 3 bunches or two bags of prepared greens)
2 teaspoons olive oil
1 medium onion, minced
6 cloves garlic, chopped
1 cup vegetable broth
1 teaspoon smoked paprika
1 teaspoon smoked salt
1 Tablespoon smoked black pepper

Instructions

- Wash greens thoroughly, removing the thick stems. Cut into 1" slices.
- In a large cast iron or heavy bottomed Dutch oven, sauté onion until soft. Add garlic, paprika, salt and pepper. Stir and cook for about 2 minutes.
- Add greens by the handful, stirring until they are coated with oil and spices, and begin to cook down (wilt).
- Once all the greens have been added to the pan, add your broth, then cover pot and simmer for about 10 minutes.
- Remove cover and cook an additional 2-5 minutes.
- Add vinegar, red pepper flakes or hot sauce at the table for an extra kick.

Fried Okra
Serves 6

Fried okra is so yummy as a snack, or served with beans and other vegetables as a side.

Ingredients

1 pound okra, sliced with tips and ends removed (about 4 cups)
Creole seasoning to taste
½ cup cornmeal
1 cup mixture of oil and Magic Vegan Bacon Grease (for frying)

Instructions

- Place cornmeal and Creole seasoning in small plastic bag.
- Add sliced okra to cornmeal and shake well until okra is well coated.
- Heat ½ cup of the oil in a heavy-bottomed skillet and fry half the okra until brown.
- Clean out pan, heat the rest of the oil and fry balance of okra.

Massaged Kale Salad
Serves 2-4

Saw a meme that said "No One Ever Got Fat From Eating Too Much Kale!" Not sure how true it is, but I do know that I love kale. Adding raw foods to your diet (especially fresh raw greens), is vital for proper vegan nutrition. This salad tastes even better a few hours later (after it's had a chance to marinate in the seasonings). I use a stick blender to mix the dressing.

Ingredients

1 large bunch of kale leaves, tough stems removed, chopped large (organic preferred)
1 ripe Hass avocado
1 Meyer lemon, juiced
2 teaspoons tamari or Bragg's aminos
2 cloves garlic, minced
½ teaspoon sea salt (or more to taste)
1 Tablespoon nutritional yeast
1½ teaspoons agave syrup
1 carrot, peeled and grated
½ cup cucumber, chopped small
6 baby Heirloom tomatoes, quartered
1 oz raw sesame seeds
Fresh ground black pepper

Instructions

- Peel avocado and remove seed. Blend avocado, lemon juice, agave, nutritional yeast, garlic, salt, and tamari together well.
- Place washed and dried kale in a large bowl. Spoon dressing onto kale, and massage into kale using both hands. Squeeze and knead the kale like you would bread.
- Continue mashing (massaging) kale for 3-4 minutes to break down tough fibers and blend flavors together. Kale will become a deep, dark green, and look slightly wilted.
- Toss in grated carrot, tomatoes, sesame seeds, and chopped cucumber; stir to mix.
- Taste and adjust seasonings if necessary before serving. Plate, then top with fresh ground black pepper.

Beer Batter Tempeh "Fish" Sticks
Serves 4

As a child I really enjoyed taking fishing and camping trips with my family. Though I no longer eat fish, I do still enjoy the taste of tartar sauce, and hush puppies or fries with a plant-based fish substitute. Enter the tempeh mock fish stick. Fire Tartar Sauce (page 21) is my favorite condiment, but malt vinegar, hot sauce, or even ketchup on the side helps make the meal complete.

Ingredients

2 packages of tempeh, cut in half

½ teaspoon kelp seasoning

2 cups chickpea flour

1 Tablespoon baking powder

1 Tablespoon garlic powder

1 Tablespoon chili powder

2 teaspoons onion powder

½ teaspoon black pepper

½ teaspoon seasoned salt

2 teaspoons Old Bay seasoning

1 Tablespoon balsamic vinegar

1 Tablespoon apple cider vinegar

1 teaspoon agave nectar or molasses

12 oz bottle of pale beer

1 cup corn or potato starch

¼ teaspoon cayenne pepper

1 Tablespoon kelp seasoning

Grape seed, peanut or canola oil (for frying)

Instructions

• Place steamer basket over pot of water. Add tempeh blocks and sprinkle with ½ tsp kelp seasoning. Steam for 10 minutes. Once cool enough to handle, cut each tempeh block into thin slices so you end up with 16 total.

• Put flour, onion and garlic powder, chili powder, pepper, salt and Old Bay seasoning into small bowl. Mix well.

• In a plastic or glass container, mix together vinegar and agave. Add to flour mixture. Slowly add beer until mixture reaches the consistency of thick pancake batter.

• In another small bowl, mix the starch and 1 rounded Tablespoon of kelp seasoning; stir well.

• Heat 3" of oil in skillet. Dredge tempeh in the starch/kelp mixture, shaking off excess, then coat with the beer batter. Be gentle, as your tempeh may start to crumble and fall apart.

- Fry the tempeh in the skillet in small batches over medium heat, turning once to brown to the other side, until golden brown all over.
- Remove the fish sticks from oil and drain on paper towels; sprinkle with salt if desired.
- Serve hot with sides such as fries, hush puppies, coleslaw or potato salad.

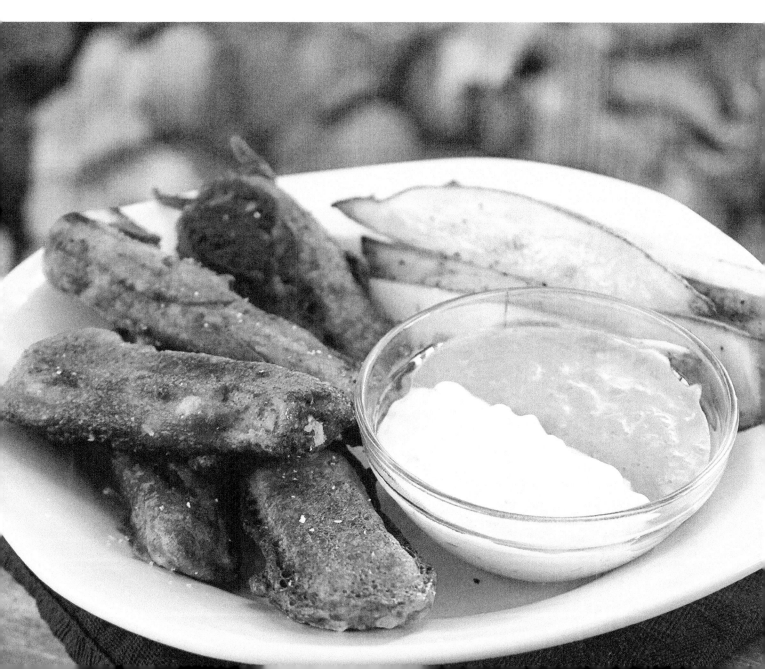

Andouille Sausage Style Seitan
Makes 8 Links

These "sausages" are meat free, 100% delicious, tender, and bring the heat. They're spicy, but not to the point of ridiculousness. They also grill up nicely and taste really good on a bun topped with Creole mustard or barbecue sauce. I use them sliced up in red beans and rice, and in jambalaya.

Ingredients

--Dry Ingredients
1½ cups vital wheat gluten
¼ cup nutritional yeast
⅓ cup chickpea flour
2 teaspoons smoked paprika
½ teaspoon black pepper
¼ teaspoon rubbed sage
½ teaspoon cayenne pepper
2 teaspoons Creole seasoning

--Wet Ingredients
½ cup water or red wine
½ cup vegetable broth
4 Tablespoons olive oil
½ cup cooked garbanzo beans
4 chipotle peppers in adobo sauce
1½ teaspoons dried thyme leaves
2 bay leaves, crumbled
1 Tablespoon lite tamari sauce
6 cloves garlic
1 teaspoon hickory smoke flavoring
1 Tablespoon raw blue agave syrup
1 not-beef bouillon cube
½ large white onion, chopped
6 dried pequin peppers

Instructions

• Put wet ingredients into food processor or blender and process until completely smooth.
• Put dry ingredients into a large bowl and whisk together to blend.
• Push dry ingredients to the side of bowl to create a valley in the center, and pour the wet ingredients into center as you mix dry with wet using rubber spatula. Scrape the sides and make sure all ingredients are blended thoroughly.
• Knead dough with fingers for 4-5 minutes until it gets tougher and firmer. Leave in bowl to rest.
• While dough rests, put steamer basket in large pot over medium heat. Make sure water

level is low enough that it doesn't come up to the steamer. This is important to avoid getting sausages wet.

- Cut 8 strips of aluminum foil that are about 6x8" square.
- Remove dough from bowl, flatten into a rectangle, and cut it into 8 even strips. Lay it on the long side of the foil and roll it up loosely (leave room for seitan to expand slightly), sealing the ends with a twist. Each one will resemble a futuristic Tootsie Roll candy.
- Stack them in the steamer basket, leaving room for steam to surround each one. Cover pot and steam for 20 minutes. Check water level and rotate top rolls to bottom.
- Return to a boil and continue steaming for another 20 minutes. Seitan should be firm to the touch in its foil casing, but not hard.
- Remove from the pan to rack with tongs and set on rack to cool.
- Refrigerate in foil wrapper in sealed plastic container or zip-style bag for up to two weeks, or freeze for up to six months.

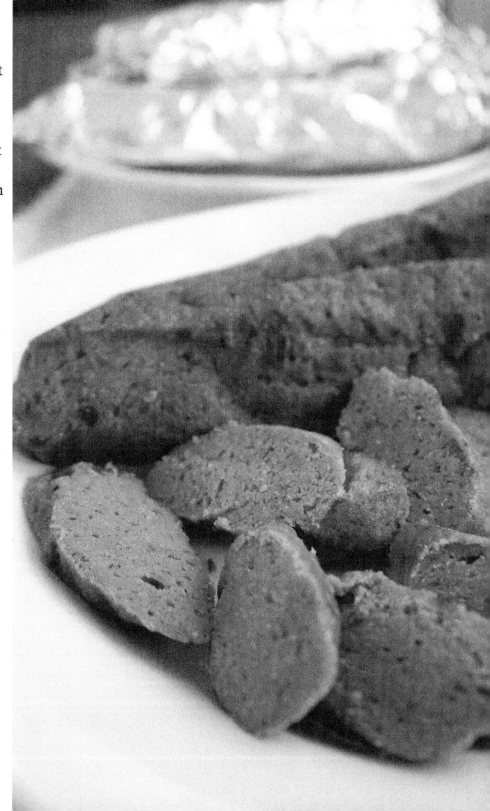

Green Lentil Sloppy Joes
Serves 6

A new twist on an old favorite, with all the same flavors.

Ingredients

1½ cups green lentils, picked over and rinsed well
4 cloves garlic
1 onion, cut in quarters
1 green bell pepper, cut in large pieces
3 Tablespoons dark brown sugar
3 Tablespoons dark molasses
1 teaspoon chili powder
1 bay leaf
3 Tablespoons tamari or Bragg's aminos
2 cups water
2 not-beef bouillon cubes
1 bottle dark beer
1 bottle full of water or vegetable broth
1 can diced tomatoes with chilies (with juice)
3 Tablespoons ketchup
1 Tablespoon olive oil
½ teaspoon seasoning salt

Instructions

- Throw onion, garlic and bell pepper in food processor. Pulse about 6-7 times until chopped. Pour into 4 quart saucepan.
- Add remaining ingredients to pan, stir well, cover and bring to boil. Once boiling, reduce heat and simmer lentils for about 30 minutes.
- Stir well, recover and simmer another 20 minutes
- Stir, taste seasonings and adjust as necessary. Remove bay leaf.
- Continue cooking with lid off for another 10 minutes or until lentils are tender.
- Spoon over hamburger buns and serve hot.

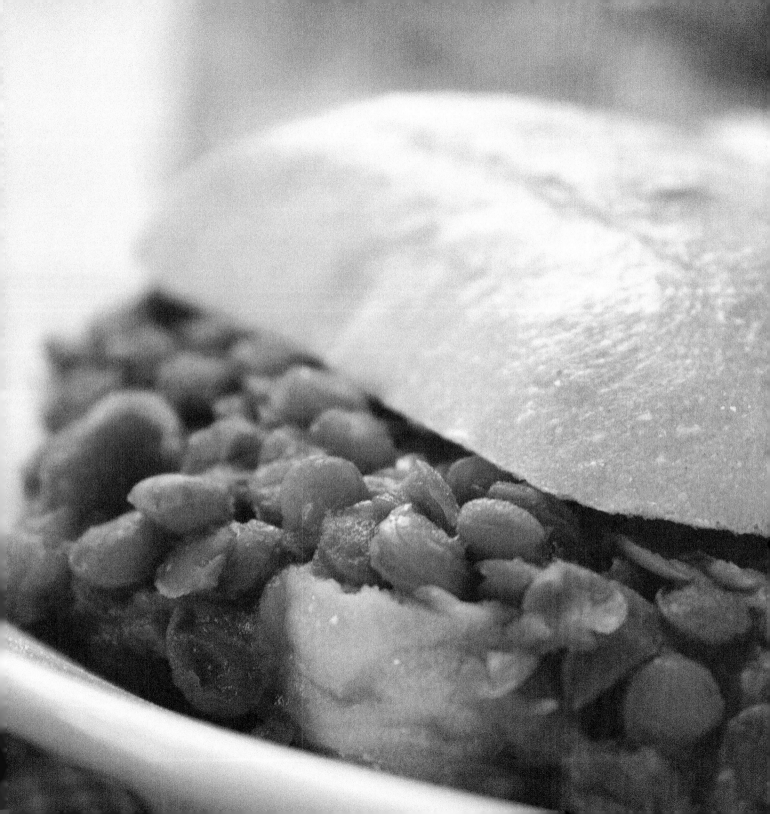

Individual Chick'n Pot Pies
Makes 6 Pies

After making a batch of chicken-style seitan, you may be wondering what to do with it. Bottom line is it can fill in as a protein source in just about any chicken dish you made in the past. Here it's combined with frozen vegetables and your favorite biscuit dough or vegan puff pastry to make delicious mini vegan "chicken" pot pies.

Ingredients

½ cup chopped celery

1 cup minced onion

2 cloves garlic

3 Tablespoons vegan butter, melted

3 Tablespoon olive oil

⅓ cup unbleached flour

3 cups hot water

2 medium potatoes, diced (1½ cups)

1 16 oz bag frozen mixed vegetables (without lima beans)

½ cup soy or almond milk

1 cup diced chicken-style seitan

1 not-chicken broth cube

2 sprigs fresh thyme

1 Tablespoon not-chicken seasoning paste

1 bay leaf

½ teaspoon each salt and pepper

Instructions

- Preheat oven to 425. Spray interior of six small foil loaf pans or 12 oz ramekins with non-stick spray.
- In a large skillet over medium heat, sauté the onions, garlic and celery in vegan butter and olive oil until soft and translucent (about 4-5 minutes).
- Stir in flour and cook for 2-3 minutes until light brown. Add water, broth cube, seasoning paste, bay leaf, salt, pepper and thyme. Let simmer for another 2-3 minutes.
- Add frozen vegetables, potato, and almond or soy milk. Cover, bring to a boil, then reduce heat and simmer until potatoes are tender, about 12 minutes.
- Turn off heat; remove thyme stems and bay leaf from pot. Stir in chopped seitan. Divide mixture between six ramekins. Then top with a bit of biscuit dough, and bake until biscuits are golden brown (about 25 minutes).

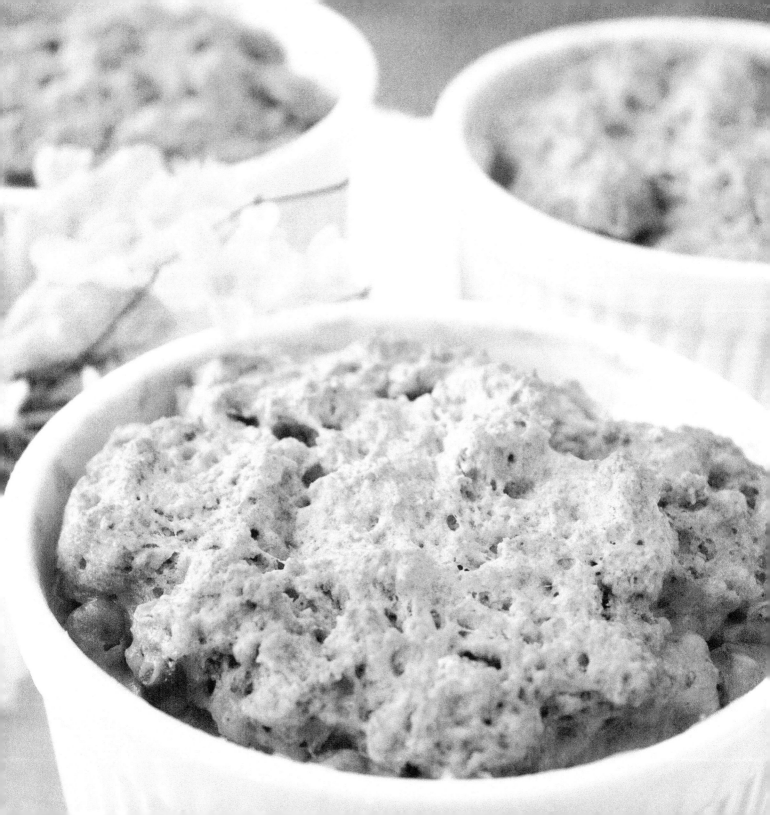

Oh Wee! Garlic Spaghetti Sauce
Serves 6-8

I've had this recipe since I was 12 years old. It was given to me by the mother of one of the members of my Girl Scout troop as we worked on our Cooking badge. Her mom was very supportive of my desire to cook cuisines of different nations, and helped by providing me with something from her Italian roots. I've learned over the years that dried herbs are convenient, but flavors are much richer if you can lay your hands on fresh basil, rosemary, parsley, thyme and oregano. The ratio for fresh to dry is 3:1, or three times as much fresh herbs as you would need if using dried. Take care to adjust the recipe accordingly.

Ingredients

3 (32 oz) cans whole plum tomatoes in juice

2 cups good quality red wine

Water as needed if sauce gets too thick

10 medium to large cloves of garlic

1 whole large yellow onion, cut into chunks

1 small whole green pepper, cut into chunks

2 stalks celery, cut into 3" pieces

12 cremini or white mushrooms

3 Tablespoons fresh oregano leaves

3 Tablespoons fresh basil leaves, chopped

1 teaspoon dried marjoram

2 teaspoons dried sage

1½ teaspoons fresh rosemary, minced

⅓ cup fresh parsley, chopped

3 Tablespoons agave nectar or sugar

1 Tablespoon fresh thyme leaves, minced

1 Tablespoon sea salt

Instructions

- Puree tomatoes and juice, vegetables and garlic in blender or food processor, 2-3 cups at a time. Add a few tablespoons of wine as needed during processing. Pour into large pot as you go.

- Add spices and salt to pot. Slowly bring to boiling, then reduce heat and simmer over low heat for 2½-3 hours, stirring regularly.

- Oh Wee! sauce is best made the day before you want to use it, as the flavors blend together and it tastes even better.

This sauce is extremely versatile and is an excellent meatless sauce for vegans and vegetarians just sprinkled with your favorite vegan Parmesan. Or you can serve it with meatless meatballs, vegan ground meat or Italian sausage product, or use it in lasagna. I've also used it as a simmer sauce for seitan "meatballs", and as a sauce for steamed vegetables.

Since it makes quite a large quantity, it's perfect for a family of mixed eaters, as the one sauce can be made then served to everyone with their own add-ins, whether omnivore or vegan.

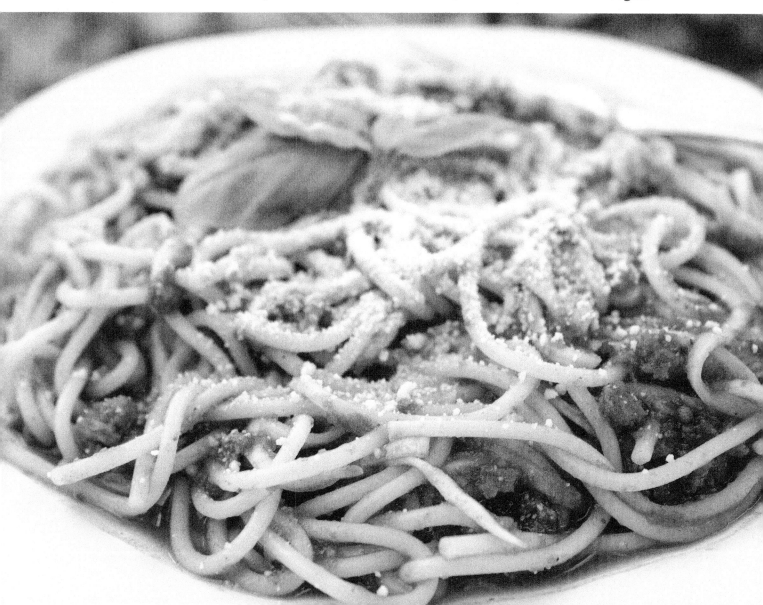

Chick'n Noodle Soup
Makes 6-8 Servings

A vegan version of the childhood comfort food favorite. Full of noodles and vegetables, this tasty soup whips up in only 15 minutes. Use whichever brand of lightly seasoned vegan "chicken" strips that you prefer.

Ingredients

2 Tablespoons olive oil

1 medium onion, diced

1 large carrot, peeled and sliced ¼" thick

1 large stalk celery, sliced ¼" thick

6 cups hot water

3 not-chicken bouillon cubes

½ teaspoon dried thyme leaves

1 bay leaf

½ package (about 1 cup) vegan chicken strips, cut into ¼" chunks

½ teaspoon salt (or to taste)

¼ cup minced fresh parsley leaves

Fresh ground black pepper

2 cups wide vegan noodles

Instructions

• Heat vegetable oil in large stock pot over med-high heat. Add onion, carrot, and celery, and sauté until softened (about 5 minutes).

• Add bay leaf, thyme leaves, water, not-chicken cubes, and minced vegan 'chicken' product). Lower heat to simmer and continue cooking until vegetables are tender.

• Add noodles and cook until tender according to package directions (usually about 5 minutes).

• Remove bay leaf; stir in minced parsley and black pepper to taste.

Crock Pot Barbecue Beans
Serves 10-12

Attending family functions when you're the only vegan can be a challenge, but if you bring something within the realm of "normal" people will happily eat your dish. These beans taste great, and can cook up the day before you need them in the crock pot. Bring a serving or two of bean burgers or seitan ribz if you'll be the only vegan in attendance.

Ingredients

1 16 oz package of dried navy beans

½ cup finely chopped onion

½ cup peeled and chopped apple chunks

8 cups of water

½ cup favorite smoky barbecue sauce

¼ cup bottled chili sauce

1 teaspoon seasoned salt

½ teaspoon dry mustard

Instructions

- Sort the beans, removing any broken or damaged ones, pebbles, etc. Rinse in fine mesh strainer and drain.

- In large pot or Dutch oven, combine the beans, onion, apple and water. Bring to a boil, then lower heat to medium.

- Cook over medium heat for 30 minutes, then remove from heat and let stand with top on for 90 minutes until beans are tender.

- Pour beans into 4 quart slow cooker. Add all remaining ingredients and stir well.

- Cover and cook on low for 9-10 hours or until beans are tender and a deep rich brown.

- Check pot while cooking and stir occasionally if needed.

Chick'n Jambalaya
Makes 6-8 Servings

A remake of a Cajun classic, something I made often to use up leftover chicken. Here chicken style seitan is used instead as the protein source, while all the same flavors and smells titillate your senses. Remember, Cajun and Creole cooking uses WHITE rice. I've never tried this with brown rice, so I cannot tell you how it will taste if you decide to use that instead. I stick with what works 'cause in my mind, if it ain't broke, don't fix it.

Ingredients

1½ lbs chick'n style seitan, cut into ½" chunks
¼ cup olive or peanut oil
3 onions, chopped
1 clove garlic
½ teaspoon white pepper
1 teaspoon Cajun or Creole seasoning salt
1 bell pepper, chopped fine
1 teaspoon thyme leaves
6 cups water
3 not-chicken broth cubes
½ teaspoon cayenne pepper
1 15 oz can chopped tomatoes
5 stalks celery, chopped fine
3 cups long grain white or Jasmine rice
½ cup chopped green onions
½ cup minced parsley
Hot pepper sauce to taste (optional)

Instructions

- Heat oil in large pot. Add chopped onions, celery and bell pepper and sauté for about five minutes.
- Mix in the garlic, thyme leaves, and tomatoes.
- Fry for a couple of minutes, then add the water, thyme, seasoning salt, white pepper and bouillon cubes. Simmer, uncovered, about 10 minutes.
- Reduce heat to low. Add the cayenne, white pepper, and seasoning salt and stir. Taste, and adjust seasonings as desired. Then stir in the rice. Cover pot and cook for 15 minutes.
- Add the chopped chick'n seitan, re-cover pot and continue to cook until the rice is tender, an additional 12-15 minutes.
- Stir in the chopped green onions and parsley. Mix well, let stand for 5-10 minutes to fluff, then serve.

Where's The Beef-y Seitan?
Serves 4-6

Most seitan recipes you'll run across are designed to substitute for chicken. That's great, but sometimes as a transitioning vegan, you'll have cravings for a "beefy" texture and flavor; this recipe meets that demand perfectly. It's extremely versatile, and can be cut up fine in a food processor and used as a ground beef substitute, or grilled as a burger. If you cook it in a broth flavored with Italian seasoning or in barbecue sauce, it will make tasty "meatballs" for pasta dishes or party snacks.

Ingredients

1 Tablespoon olive oil
1 teaspoon vegan Worcestershire sauce
1 Tablespoon Montreal steak seasoning
1 cup water
6 cremini mushrooms, cleaned removed
2 shallots, cut in half
1 clove garlic
10 fresh basil leaves
1 cup vital wheat gluten
2 Tablespoons nutritional yeast flakes
2 Tablespoons chickpea flour
1 teaspoon non-aluminum baking powder

--For Simmering Broth

1 bay leaf
6 black peppercorns
½ teaspoon Apple wood or hickory liquid smoke flavoring

5 cups water
1 onion, sliced
1 carrot, chopped
1 Tablespoon parsley
1 teaspoon red pepper flakes
3 Tablespoons tamari
1 not-beef seasoning cube

Instructions

- Combine olive oil, Worcestershire sauce, tamari and water in food processor with mushrooms, shallots, garlic and basil. Process until smooth.
- In large mixing bowl, measure out wheat gluten, chickpea flour, baking powder and yeast flakes. Blend well.
- Slowly pour liquid ingredients into dry ingredients, mixing with rubber spatula.

Instructions (continued)

- Dough will quickly form a ball. Mix and press dry ingredients into ball with spatula until all dry ingredients are incorporated.
- Remove dough from bowl and knead for 3-4 minutes, then return to bowl. Let rest while you prepare the simmering broth.
- Mix all the broth ingredients together into large stock pot.
- Divide dough into 8 pieces for burger or "steak" patties, or small pieces for "meatballs." Burger patties should be flattened to no more than ¼" in thickness (they will double in size when cooking. Really stretch them out! Don't be afraid to tear a hole in the dough, as it will fill in as the dough cooks.
- Once you've shaped all the patties, put them in the cold broth, cover, then turn heat to medium. Once it gets close to boiling, reduce heat to slow simmer and cook for 30 minutes.
- Remove pot from heat and let seitan cool with broth in pan. If you will not be cooking all your seitan, be sure to store it in the broth for maximum flavor and to preserve juiciness.
- If you are going to cook it right away, once broth cools, remove seitan onto plate or rack to drain, then do your thing.

Note:
Feel free to add a few Tablespoons of dry red wine to your simmering broth for a richer flavor experience.

Sweets, Treats & Desserts

Sweet Potato & Parsnip Cupcakes
Makes 1 Dozen

I walked by what looked to me to be bleached carroty looking things called parsnips for at least 25 years before I dared to try one. Afterwards, I wanted to kick myself for being leery of a delicious, highly versatile root vegetable. Here they're paired with sweet potatoes for a surprisingly decadent vegan dessert.

Ingredients

1 cup unbleached all-purpose flour
½ teaspoon ground cardamom
½ teaspoon ground allspice
¼ teaspoon ground nutmeg
1½ teaspoons aluminum free baking powder
¼ teaspoon Himalayan pink salt
½ cup packed brown sugar
2 egg replacer "eggs"
4 Tablespoons vegan butter, melted and Blended with oil to make total of ⅔ cup
1 cup grated parsnip
1 cup grated sweet potato

---Cream Cheeze Frosting
1 8 oz carton vegan cream cheese
4 Tablespoons vegan butter
½ cup confectioners sugar
1 teaspoon lemon extract

Instructions

- Preheat oven to 350 degrees.
- Prepare your vegan egg mixture in a small bowl in accordance with package directions.
- Melt vegan butter and stir in vegetable oil.
- Whisk together the dry ingredients in a large bowl. Add vegan egg and oils, and mix thoroughly. Stir in grated sweet potato and parsnip.
- Line muffin pan with paper liners, then carefully fill each one about ¾ full.
- Bake about 20 minutes until the top springs back when lightly pressed. Let cool on rack.
- Prepare the frosting by whipping ingredients together until fluffy. Divide evenly amongst the 12 cooled cupcakes.
- Store in refrigerator in airtight container up to two days, but they probably won't last that long.

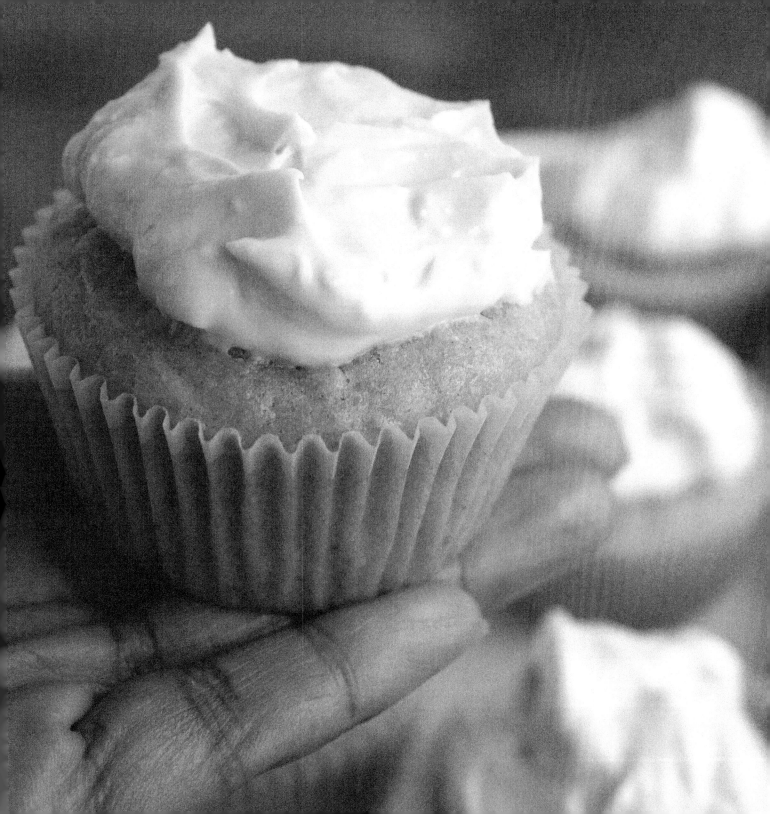

Oatmeal Shortbread Cookies
Makes About 50 Cookies

Quick to make, these rich and buttery cookies are perfect with a cup of hot coffee or your favorite non-dairy "ice cream." They're not overly sweet and children love them. Every time I take them to a potluck or party, they go fast.

Ingredients

2 vegan buttery baking sticks

¾ cup raw sugar

1½ cups all purpose flour

1½ cups quick-cooking oats

¾ teaspoon sea salt

Instructions

- Preheat oven to 325 degrees.
- Cream butter and sugar together with mixer until light and fluffy.
- Gradually add the flour, oats and salt.
- Press with fingertips into a greased 13x9" baking pan.
- Prick dough with a fork a few times in several places (helps keep the cookies flat).
- Bake for 30-35 minutes or until lightly browned.
- Cool for 10 minutes before cutting into small rectangular bars or squares. Depending upon the size you cut, you should have between 40-60 cookies.

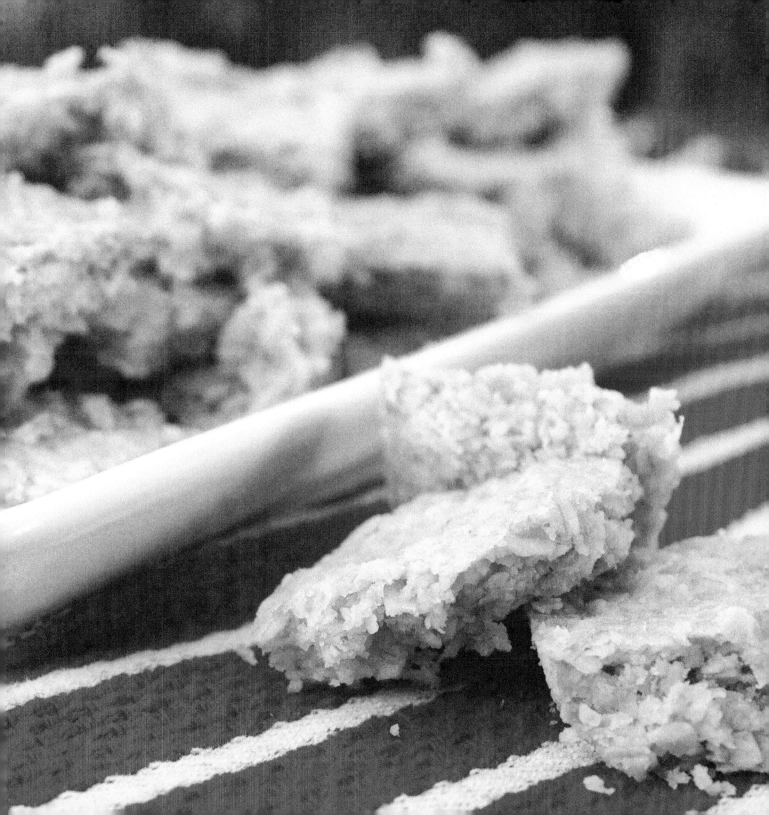

Cashew Crunch Cookies
Makes 60 Cookies

Not sure where I got this recipe from, but it's written in my teen curlicue style handwriting, which means it must have been something I liked enough to ask the maker for the recipe.

Ingredients

2¼ cups all purpose unbleached flour

½ teaspoon baking soda

½ teaspoon cream of tartar

¾ cup firmly packed brown sugar

1 teaspoon vanilla extract

½ cup sugar

1 cup soft vegan butter

1 vegan "egg"

1½ cups finely chopped cashews

Instructions

• Preheat oven to 350 degrees.

• In large mixing bowl, combine all the ingredients (except cashews). Blend well with mixer.

• Stir in cashews by hand, mixing thoroughly.

• Drop by rounded teaspoons onto lightly greased cookie sheet.

• Bake for 12-15 minutes or until golden brown.

Chickpea & Chips Cookies
Makes 2 Dozen

One of my personal training clients gave this recipe a few years ago when she found out I liked chickpea everything. They're gluten free, dairy free and easy to make. These cookies do not get firm like flour-based cookies, they will remain soft. They're best warm, so keep the dough in the refrigerator and make only the number you plan to eat right away.

Ingredients

1¼ cups canned chickpeas (garbanzo beans), drained, rinsed and patted dry

2 teaspoons vanilla extract

½ cup plus 2 Tablespoons non-commercial (natural) peanut or almond butter, at room temperature

¼ cup pure maple syrup

1 teaspoon aluminum free baking powder

½ cup vegan semi-sweet chocolate chips

¼ teaspoon of salt (if using unsalted nut butter)

‡ Vegan brands of chocolate chips are sold at Whole Foods, Trader Joe's, most health food stores, or can be ordered through online retailers.

Instructions

• Preheat oven to 350 degrees.

• Combine chickpeas, vanilla, nut butter, maple syrup, and baking powder in food processor. Scrape sides as needed and blend until mixture is very smooth.

• Stir in chocolate chips by hand. The mixture will be very gooey and sticky!

• Roll pinches of dough into 1" ball. Place them on an ungreased cookie sheet.

• Press down lightly so balls are slightly flattened rounds.

• Bake for 10 minutes. Remove pan from oven and cool cookies on baking sheet for 10 minutes before removing them from pan.

Fresh Peach Cobbler
Serves 12

This is my paternal grandmother's recipe for cobbler, which is the only one I will eat. To me, canned peaches result in a pan full of mushy, overcooked peaches with crust. "Ma dear" would only make cobbler when peaches were in season, and it was the best! Warm from the oven and topped with heavy cream, it was delicious, but I've replaced dairy with whipped coconut cream.

Ingredients

4 pounds fresh peaches, peeled and sliced

1½ cups sugar

½ cup flour

½ cup cold water

4 Tablespoons vegan butter

2 teaspoons ground nutmeg

2 teaspoons vanilla extract

--- Cobbler Crust

2 cups all purpose unbleached flour

2 teaspoons baking powder

¾ teaspoon salt

1 stick vegan buttery spread

⅔ cup ice cold water

Instructions

- Preheat oven to 375 degrees.
- In a large saucepan combine sliced peaches and sugar. Let stand while you make your crust.
- Whisk flour, baking powder, and salt together. Cut in vegan butter until fine crumbs form. Gradually blend in the cold water with a fork. Turn onto a well-floured board; knead until smooth and stickiness disappears. Roll out a 9x13" rectangle.
- Blend ½ cup water and flour together until smooth. Stir into peach/sugar mixture.
- Cook peaches over med-low heat, stirring frequently, until mixture boils and thickens. Stir in the vegan butter, nutmeg and vanilla extract, then pour into baking dish.
- Arrange dough over fruit. Make slashes in top and sprinkle with sugar. Bake until crust is golden brown, about 45 minutes.

Whipped Coconut Cream Topping
Makes 2 Cups

None of the dairy fat or hormones, and all of the rich flavor of a decadent whipped cream topping. Use coconut cream topping on pies, cakes, cupcakes, or cobblers.

Ingredients

1 8 oz carton or can of coconut cream

1-2 Tablespoons confectioners sugar

Instructions

• Chill unopened carton of coconut cream in refrigerator for a few hours or overnight.

• Pour into chilled mixing bowl and beat with an immersion blender for about 5 minutes, or until coconut cream is thick and fluffy.

• Add in the powdered sugar and beat another 20-30 seconds.

• Place container in the refrigerator for 5-10 minutes to firm whipped cream before use.

Coconut Oil Pie Crust
Makes Two Crusts

Though my grandmother would be appalled, using a food processor to whip up this pie crust makes it fast and easy, and it's still flaky and delicious. Use it to replace pie crusts made with lard or hydrogenated shortening. This recipe make two pies, one pie with a double crust, or one large (deep dish) pie with a lattice style top crust. Freeze leftovers in zip style freezer bag.

Ingredients

2¼ cups all purpose flour

½ cup plus 2 Tablespoons coconut oil

(measured in solid state, chilled)

1 teaspoon sea salt

1 Tablespoon cane sugar

½ cup ice cold water

Instructions

- Put dry ingredients in the food processor and pulse a few times to blend. Add chilled coconut oil and pulse until mixture resembles fine meal.
- Start slowly pouring in cold water - begin with ⅓ cup, adding more by the Tablespoon until mixture starts to form a ball in the food processor.
- Turn dough out onto well-floured counter or board, and divide in half.
- Flip to coat with flour on both sides, then roll out until it's about 2" larger than your pie pan. Add additional flour as needed to prevent sticking.
- Fold pie crust in half, then over again to form a ¼ wedge slice. Place in pie pan and unfold. Pinch edges to form a ridge. Keep crust in refrigerator until filling is prepared.

Aunt Emma's Cheesecake Cookies
Makes 1 Dozen

Another find from my cruddy looking recipe box - the one I've had for almost 40 years. My mom's youngest sister and my favorite aunt (Aunt Emma), made these often when I'd visit during the summer to tutor my grade school cousins.

Ingredients

1 cup all purpose flour

⅓ cup vegan butter, softened

⅓ cup firmly packed light brown sugar

½ cup chopped walnuts

8 oz carton vegan cream cheese

¼ cup sugar

1 vegan "egg"

2 Tablespoons almond milk

2 Tablespoons fresh lemon juice

½ teaspoon vanilla extract

Instructions

- Preheat oven to 350 degrees.
- In a large mixing bowl, combine the flour, butter and brown sugar. Blend with electric mixer until fine particles form. Stir in the chopped walnuts. Reserve 1 cup of this mixture for the topping.
- Press remainder of mix into ungreased 8x8" square baking pan. Bake for 12-15 minutes, or until lightly browned.
- In the same bowl, combine the remaining ingredients. Blend well, then spread over partially baked crust. Sprinkle with reserved crumb mixture.
- Return pan to oven and bake another 25-30 minutes.
- Cool on wire rack and cut into 12-15 squares.
- Store uneaten cookies in the refrigerator.

Chia Seed Pudding
Serves 3-4

Chia seeds are a rich source of Omega-3 fats (even better than flax seeds), plus they're super high in antioxidants, fiber, calcium, magnesium, niacin and zinc. With a nut-like flavor and the ability to "gel" when added to water, chia makes a nutritious and tasty pudding-like dessert.

Ingredients

2 cups vanilla flavored almond milk

3 Tablespoons pure maple syrup

1 teaspoon vanilla extract

½ cup chia seeds

Instructions

- Whisk together maple syrup, almond milk and vanilla extract.
- Stir in the chia seeds. Let mixture gel for 10 minutes. Then stir again.
- Place in refrigerator to chill for 4-5 hours (or overnight) before serving.
- Serve chilled or at room temperature, topped with berries, ground or chopped nuts, currants, chopped dates, cranberries, or a dollop of whipped coconut cream topping.

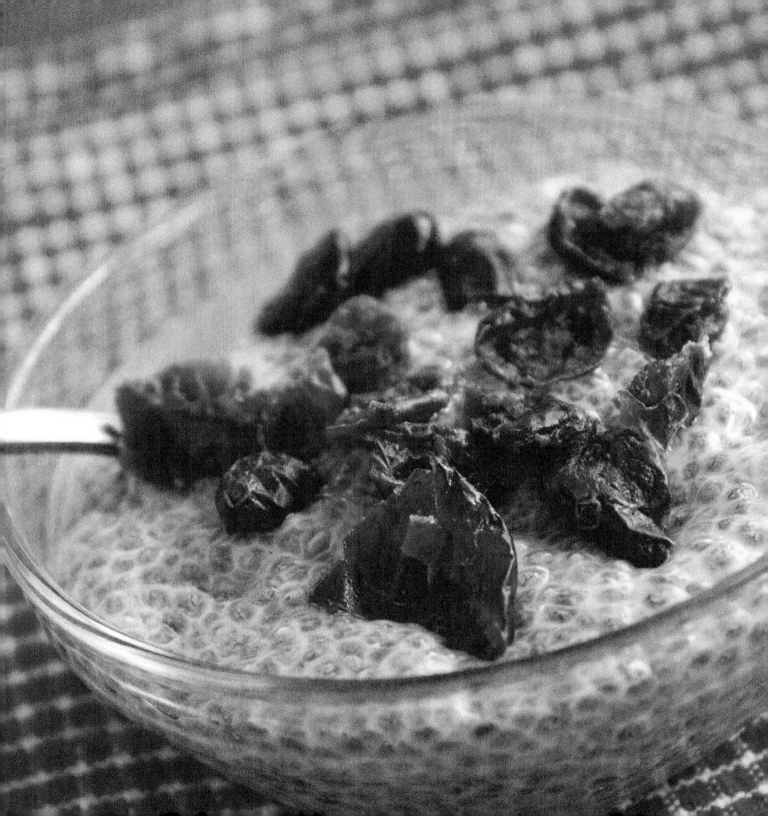

Spiced Apple Betty
Serves 6

From my Mom - a fabulous summertime dessert that's lighter and faster to make than a cobbler. Try it with other in season fruit such as peaches, pears, apples, or apricots.

Ingredients

2 cups fresh diced apples

1 cup packed dark brown sugar

1 cup all purpose flour

⅛ teaspoon ground nutmeg

¼ teaspoon ground cinnamon

½ cup (1 stick) vegan butter plus

2 Tablespoons vegan butter for pan

Instructions

• Preheat oven to 350 degrees.

• Peel and chop apples and place in buttered 8x8" square baking dish.

• Mix dry ingredients together. Cut in butter with pastry blender and sprinkle over apples.

• Bake for about 40 minutes, until topping is a nice toasty brown.

Broke Folks Cake
Serves 8-10

Evidently this type of cake was very common during the Great Depression and World War II, when it was a challenge to get your hands on luxury items like baking powder or fresh eggs unless you lived on a farm. As a child I didn't know anything about that, I just knew that my grandmother made it often and it tasted good.

Ingredients

2 cups sugar

1 Tablespoon vegan buttery spread

1 pound of raisins

2 teaspoons salt

2 teaspoons ground cinnamon

1 teaspoon ground nutmeg

2¾ cups water

2 teaspoons baking soda

2 teaspoons water

4 cups all purpose unbleached flour

Instructions

- Grease and flour a Bundt pan. Sit it to the side.
- Boil sugar, buttery spread, raisins, cinnamon, salt, nutmeg and water together in a large pot for 5 minutes. Remove from heat and cool for 45 minutes.
- Dissolve baking soda in 2 teaspoons of water, stir well then add it to the pot and stir.
- Remove from pot to bowl; add flour, about ½ cup at a time, until thoroughly blended. You'll need to use some muscle because the batter will be very thick. Spoon into your prepared Bundt pan and bake at 300 degrees for about 90 minutes.
- When done cake should spring back when touched, and a toothpick inserted near the center should come back clean.
- Cool then slice.

BaChocButter Ice Cream
Serves 2

You can thank my picky five year old cousin for the name of this frozen dessert. I was attempting to get some extra protein into the child (she eats like a bird), and came up with this. We used something called PB2 in chocolate flavor, and sprinkled a few vegan chocolate chips and chopped walnuts on it for visual appeal. Sorry, no pictures. Burp.

Ingredients

2 ripe organic bananas, peeled and frozen

2-3 Tablespoons chilled vanilla almond milk

2-3 Tablespoons peanut protein powder in chocolate flavor

2 Tablespoons Vegan chocolate chips (optional)

2 Tablespoons chopped walnuts (toasted) (optional)

Instructions

• Stick almond milk in the freezer for about 10 minutes to make sure it's really cold.

• Place frozen bananas and chilled almond milk into high powered blender or food processor. Add peanut protein powder.

• Pulse to break up bananas, then blend until smooth and creamy like soft serve ice cream.

• Remove from container and divide into two serving dishes. Top with toasted chopped walnuts and/or vegan chocolate chips, if desired.

• Serve immediately.

Snacks, Dips, Spreads & Appetizers

Roasted Chickpea Popcorn
Serves 4

When you want something crunchy and spicy, roasted chickpeas make a perfect snack. The seasonings suggested here are just that - suggestions. Use whatever you have on hand, in whatever quantity your palate can handle them. Ideas are cumin, chili powder, Cajun seasoning, lemon pepper seasoning, onion powder, etc.

Ingredients

2 cans (4 cups) chickpeas, rinsed and drained

3 Tablespoons olive oil

2 teaspoons garlic salt

2 teaspoons paprika

2 teaspoons cayenne pepper

2 teaspoons nutritional yeast

1 teaspoon fresh ground black pepper

Instructions

- Preheat oven to 450 degrees.
- Dump the drained chickpeas on a clean absorbent towel, and fold towel over chickpeas to absorb last bits of moisture.
- Spread chickpeas on a rimmed baking tray, then drizzle with olive oil. Roll chickpeas around with your hands to evenly coat them with oil.
- Mix seasonings together in a cup, then sprinkle evenly over chickpeas. You may need to shake the pan to redistribute the seasonings if you see spices are too heavy in some areas and light in others.
- Bake in hot oven for 25-30 minutes until lightly brown and crunchy, shaking the pan halfway to "roll" the chickpeas.
- Let them cool to warm before eating to avoid burning your mouth.

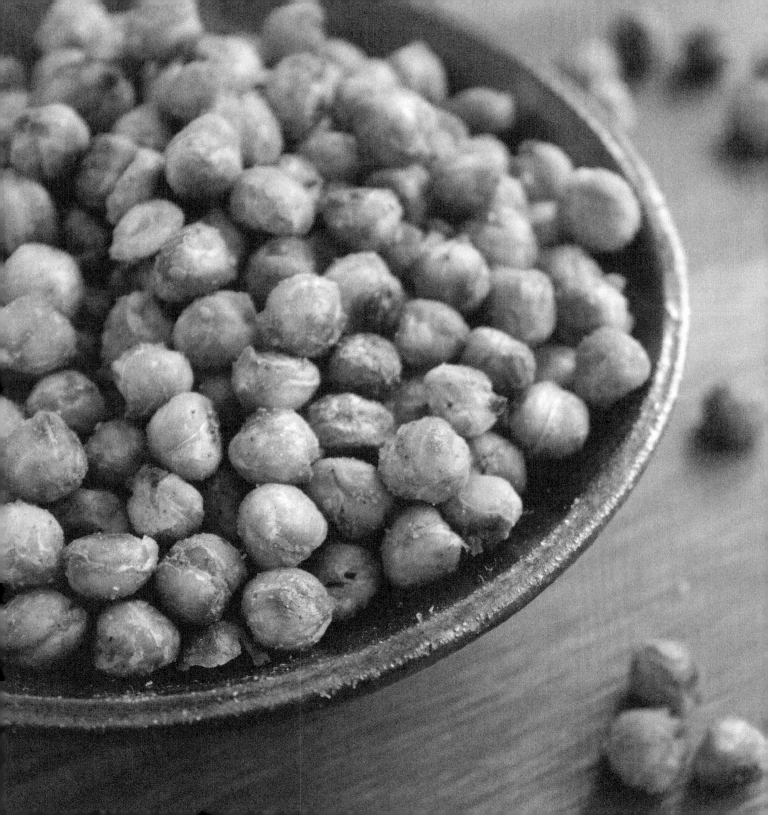

Fresh & Fonky Salsa Dip
Makes 3 Cups

The Mission District of San Francisco is full of the flavors of South America. Restaurants featuring the smells and fresh flavors of the cuisines of Mexico, Venezuela, Bolivia, Ecuador, Columbia and Brazil are common and popular. Feel free to add Mexican-style hot sauce or a diced jalapeño to increase the heat if you like your food spicy.

Ingredients

1½ tomatoes, chopped into ½" chunks

2 Tablespoons diced green chilies

1 green onion, diced

¼ green bell pepper, diced

1 Tablespoon fresh lemon juice

2 Tablespoons cilantro, chopped

1 clove garlic, minced

¼ cup tomato sauce

Pinch of fresh ground black pepper

Instructions

- Pour tomato sauce into blender.
- Combine the remaining ingredients in bowl.
- Scoop out ½ cup of onion/pepper mixture and puree in blender with tomato sauce.
- Add puree mix to salsa mixture, stir well and chill 5-6 hours (overnight is preferred).
- Serve with tortilla chips. Guacamole is nice as well.

Texas Cashew Cheeze with Hot Peppers
Makes 1 ½ Cups

My friends love spicy food. With the crew coming over for game and movie night, I was looking for something with a bit of kick, and which would provide a more interesting flavor medley for a pasta topping or Canapés (since I hadn't decided on what I was going to serve). This peppery blend (which uses fresh grapefruit and hot peppers - both from Texas), was a big hit.

Ingredients

1 cup raw cashews

½ cup water

¼ cup nutritional yeast flakes

1 Texas pink grapefruit, juiced

2 small cloves garlic

6 dried chili Pequin peppers

1 teaspoon spicy brown or Dijon mustard

1 Tablespoon sun dried tomatoes slices

Instructions

• Soak cashews in ½ cup water for about an hour. Drain and rinse in mesh strainer.

• Pack sun dried tomatoes into Tablespoon, pressing out excess oil if using oil packed.

• Add drained cashews and 4 Tablespoons of pink grapefruit juice to blender or food processor, and mix on high until smooth and creamy (about 60 seconds). Add a teaspoon more of juice if mixture is too thick.

• Remove from blender and put in airtight container. Chill several hours to overnight to allow flavors to blend before serving. Cheeze will thicken slightly.

• Great on crackers or with raw/lightly steamed veggies.

• Store unused portion in airtight container in refrigerator for up to 5 days.

Seitan Barbecued Ribz
Serves 6-8

After trying a couple of seitan rib recipes I found on the web, I developed one that tasted more like what I wanted in a rib. Be sure to let them bake or grill until the barbecue sauce becomes crispy and caramelized. You want your ribz to be fully cooked, firm, and well-seasoned – not doughy or rubbery.

Ingredients

3 cups vital wheat gluten
2 teaspoons smoked paprika
2 Tablespoons nutritional yeast flakes
2 teaspoons onion powder
½ teaspoon black pepper
1 teaspoon sea salt
1½ cups low sodium vegetable broth or water
2 Tablespoons crushed garlic
3 Tablespoons natural peanut butter (or other nut butter)
2 Tablespoons vegan butter
2 Tablespoons liquid aminos
2 Tablespoons liquid smoke
4 cups smoky barbecue sauce

Instructions

- In a large bowl, whisk together vital wheat gluten, paprika, nutritional yeast, salt, and pepper.
- In a small mixing bowl, mix butter, aminos, broth (or water), peanut butter, and garlic with stick blender until smooth.
- Add 2 cups of smoky barbecue sauce and liquid smoke to wet mixture.
- Slowly pour wet ingredients into dry while stirring with rubber spatula. Finish mixing with hands, incorporating all dry ingredients.
- Knead for 3 minutes; let rest 20-30 minutes.
- Preheat the oven to 350. Spray a 13"x9" baking dish with non-stick spray.
- Press mixture into oiled baking pan until it is flat and fills the pan. Using a sharp knife, cut the seitan about ¾ of the way through into ¾" wide "ribz".

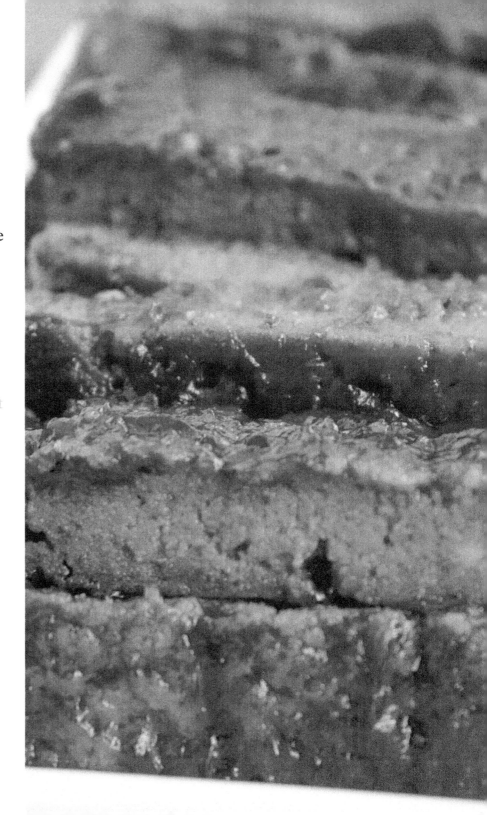

- Bake for 30 minutes, then add 1 cup or more of barbecue sauce, spreading over ribz evenly. Continue baking for another 15 minutes.
- Flip ribz over, and slather in more barbecue sauce. Bake another 20 minutes or until sauce caramelizes and turns a crispy brown on the edges and top of ribz.

‡ If you prefer to grill your ribz, after they cook about 30-40 minutes in the oven, pull them out and place them on a grill. Baste with sauce and grill for 5 minutes. Baste frequently with sauce as you turn the ribz over every 4-5 minutes for 15-20 minutes until done.

Vegan Vietnamese Spring Rolls
Serves 8-10

Try this recipe for a delicious 100% cruelty free version of the traditional crispy Vietnamese Spring Roll, with a bit of Thai influence. You'll end up with a crunchy appetizer full of nutritious shredded vegetables. Dip it in the spicy sauce for extra flavor.

Ingredients

1 package of your favorite meat substitute, ground in food processor
1 8 oz. package of mung bean noodles (or glass or cellophane noodles)
1½ cups shredded carrots
1½ cups shredded cabbage
½ cup dried black fungus strips (soaked and drained)
1 large shallot, minced
2 cloves garlic, minced
½ teaspoon vegan chicken-style seasoning
1 teaspoon fresh ground black pepper
½ teaspoon white pepper
1 teaspoon vegan fish sauce
1 teaspoon agave nectar
2 Tablespoons low sodium soy sauce
¼ teaspoon sesame oil
1 package frozen spring roll wrappers, thawed
1 flax egg (1 Tablespoon flax meal in 2 Tablespoons water)
4 cups of peanut or grape seed oil

Instructions

- Place the noodles in a large bowl and cover with warm water. Let sit and soften for 20-30 minutes, turning over halfway if needed.
- Combine the white and black pepper, soy sauce, agave and vegan fish sauce in a large bowl. Add in the ground meat replacement, and stir well.
- Once the noodles are softened, drain the water off, then cut the noodles into short pieces about 1-2" long, and drop them into the bowl.
- Add in the shredded carrots, garlic, and shallot. Stir to blend.
- Add the presoaked and drained dry fungus strips and the sesame oil. Mix everything together well.
- Remove one wrapper from the packaging and lay it on a tray. Spoon a rounded Tablespoon full of the filling mixture onto one corner of

the wrapper, then fold wrapper twice to form a triangle shape, then close both ends and tighten.

- Roll the wrapper to the end and seal it with a dab of the flax egg. Sit it on a clean, dry platter. Repeat process until you've used all your filling mixture.
- Heat peanut oil in a deep pan over medium heat. Once oil is hot, add a few spring rolls at a time to the oil and fry both sides until roll is a nice golden brown all over.
- Using a strainer basket or slotted spoon, remove the rolls from the oil, and sit them on a paper towel covered cooling rack to drain the excess oil.
- Keep warm in oven until all rolls are cooked and you're ready to serve.

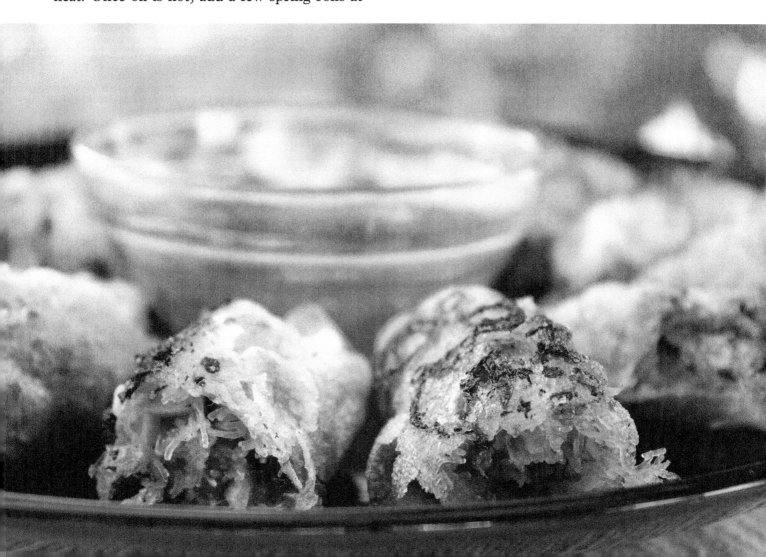

The Real Deal Nacho Dip
Makes 1½ Cups

This party dip is so filling. Be sure you have some sturdy chips for people to scoop with or you'll end up with a big mess on your hands.

Ingredients

1 package vegan "ground beef" crumbles

1 medium onion, finely chopped

1 package taco seasoning mix

⅔ cup water

1 can vegan refried beans

1 (2 oz) can diced green chilies

2 cups vegan Monterey Jack or cheddar cheeze shreds

1 cup salsa

---Garnishes

4 Tablespoons chopped green onion

1 cup sliced olives

2 ripe avocados, peeled and chopped

1 8 oz carton vegan sour cream

1 8 oz container pico de gallo

Instructions

- In a medium sized frying pan, combine water and taco seasoning mix. Bring to simmer and let thicken. Add "beef" crumbles and remove from heat.
- Spread beans evenly over the bottom of an 8x8" pan. Top beans with crumble mixture, spreading evenly.
- Layer shredded cheeze shreds across crumbles mixture as evenly as possible. Drizzle salsa over cheeze.
- Bake, uncovered, at 400 degrees for 20 minutes, or until hot throughout.
- Remove pan from oven. Garnish with green onions, olives, avocado, pico de gallo, and vegan sour cream.
- Serve with tortilla chips.

Jalapeño Chile Cheeze Dip
Makes 1½ Cups

A spicy blend of peppers and chilies that works well for enchiladas, as a dip for vegetables or tortilla chips, in cheeze quesadillas, burritos or tacos, or as a spread on sandwiches. I've even used it in tofu scrambles. This recipe is a good, flavorful alternative to pepper jack style dairy cheese.

Ingredients

½ cup raw cashews, soaked 4 hours in water

1 cup vegetable broth

1 (or more) cups water

2 Tablespoons Sriracha pepper sauce

1 Tablespoon olive oil

¼ cup nutritional yeast flakes

1 teaspoon sea salt

1 jalapeño pepper, seeded and trimmed

1 4 oz can diced green chilies, drained

Instructions

- Drain the cashews, then add them to a blender or food processor with vegetable broth. Process on high for 1 minute until smooth.

- Add remaining ingredients (except can of green chilies) to blender, and process until well combined and smooth. Add additional water as needed to keep consistency like heavy cream.

- Pour from blender into saucepan and cook over medium heat, stirring frequently, until mixture thickens.

- Remove from heat and stir in green chilies. Let cool to room temperature then serve, or place in airtight container and store in refrigerator until ready to use.

Tofu "Buffalo" Wangz
Serves 3-4

Watch out, these puppies are yummy. Devout meat eating friends - folks who turn their noses up at anything vegan or vegetarian - tore into them like no tomorrow. Use vacuum packed tofu, or press water-packed tofu dry by wrapping it in several paper towels and sitting a heavy book on it for about 30 minutes. Change the paper toweling after 10-15 minutes if it gets soaked.

Ingredients

1 15-ounce block extra firm organic tofu, (dry packed without water)
⅓ cup corn starch
½ teaspoon Himalayan pink salt
1 teaspoon garlic powder
1 teaspoon onion powder
1 teaspoon mustard powder
1 teaspoon ground black pepper
½ teaspoon cayenne pepper
½ teaspoon paprika
3 Tablespoons peanut oil for pan-frying
3 carrots, sliced into 3" sticks
3 stalks celery, sliced lengthwise then quarters

For the Sauce
¼ cup vegan buttery spread (melted measure)
⅓ cup Franks hot wing sauce
1 teaspoon agave nectar
Dash salt

Instructions

• Slice tofu into 12 or more thin rectangles, cubes, triangles, or whatever shape you like.
• Place the corn starch and spices in a plastic bag. Gently add the tofu, carefully shaking bag to make sure that all sides of the tofu is well coated with the corn starch mixture.
• Heat the oil in a large non-stick sauté pan over medium heat. Add tofu and pan-fry on all sides just until lightly golden brown. Once the tofu has cooked, remove it from the pan and drain it on paper towels.
• Place the vegan butter in the pan over a very low setting. Once melted, add the wing sauce and agave nectar, stirring just until combined.
• Heat about 2 minutes, then add the cooked tofu shapes, spooning sauce over tofu to coat it on all sides with the sauce. Be gentle to avoid breaking tofu apart.
• Gently remove tofu from pan and place on serving plate.

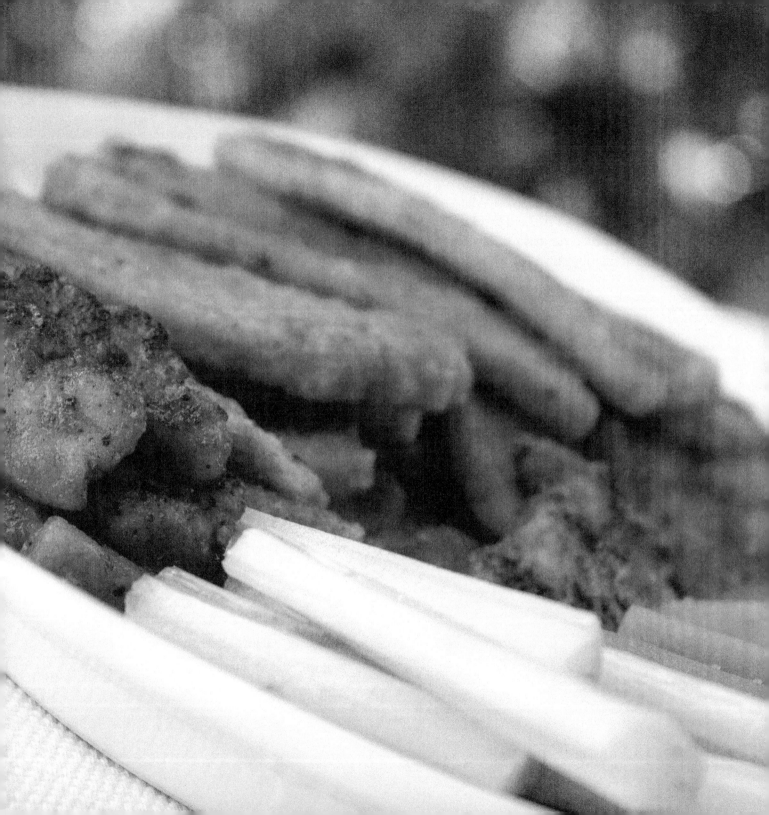

Black Bean Quesadillas
Serves 6

Make good use of your leftover spicy or Cuban-style black beans. If you have a crowd coming over you'd do well to make a triple batch of these, because they go fast. Top with store bought or home made pico de gallo salsa, vegan sour cream, sliced jalapeños, and sliced avocado or guacamole. A delicious snack or appetizer that no one will question as being vegan.

Ingredients

2 cups leftover black beans

12 8-inch artisan corn and whole grain tortillas

1 cup vegan Mexican-style cheeze strips

3 Tablespoons olive oil (divided)

Instructions

- Mix cheese strips into black beans, lightly mashing some of the beans.
- Add 1-2 teaspoons of oil to large non-stick skillet and heat over medium.
- Spread ⅓ cup of the bean mixture onto a tortilla and place in pan. Spread around with back of spoon to distribute evenly. Place second tortilla on top.
- Cook until tortilla is browned and crispy, then flip it over with a large spatula and brown second side.
- Remove from pan and cut into six pie-shaped wedges with pizza cutter or very sharp knife.
- Serve hot, garnished with avocado, pico de gallo, sliced jalapeño and/or vegan sour cream.

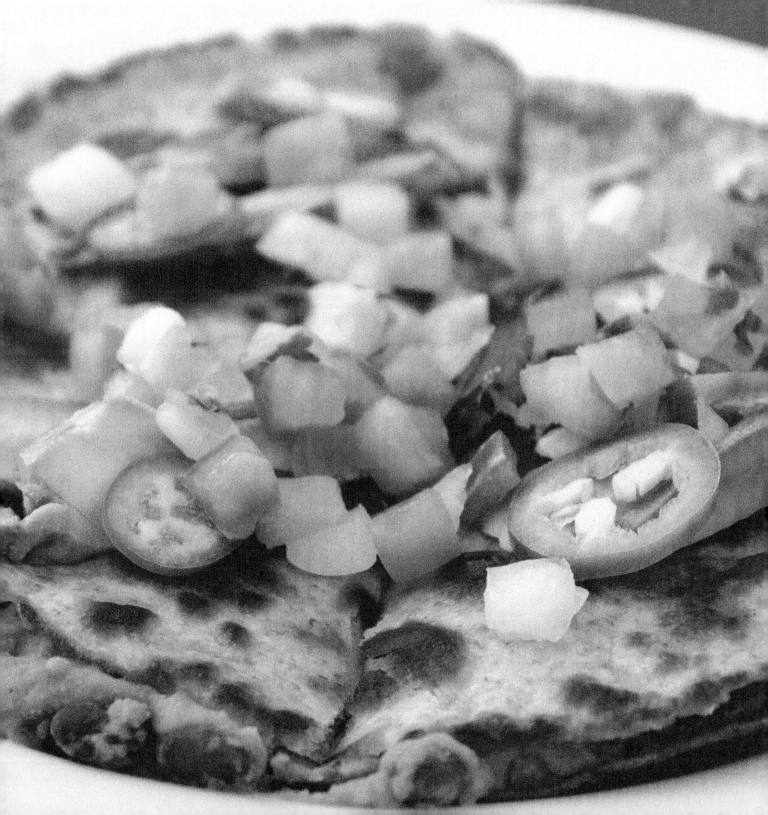

Chickpea & Veggie Sliders
Makes 20

At this point you're probably thinking "does this woman ever get tired of All Things Chickpea?" Well the answer is "nope." These little mini-veggie burgers not only taste great, they deliver a host of minerals, fiber, and protein without fat or cholesterol. Recipe makes about 20 3" slider patties or 5-6 full sized burgers. I love to serve them with peppery arugula and sliced tomato.

Ingredients

1 can organic chickpeas, rinsed and drained

2 teaspoons olive or grape seed oil

1 large white onion, quartered and sliced thin

¼ red bell pepper, chopped

1 Serrano or jalapeño, seeded and chopped

4 cloves garlic

1 cup baby carrots, chopped

2 teaspoons Creole seasoning salt, divided

1 teaspoon ground cumin

1 teaspoon curry powder or paprika

½ teaspoon ground coriander

½ teaspoon fresh ground black pepper

¼ teaspoon cayenne pepper

2 teaspoons dried thyme leaves

2 Tablespoons dried parsley leaves

1 cup panko bread crumbs

4 "eggs" made from vegan egg replacer

Instructions

- Measure out spices (1 teaspoon seasoning salt and all other spices) into cup and set aside.
- Add oil to large skillet over medium-high heat. Add onion, bell pepper, jalapeño and 1 teaspoon of seasoning salt. Cook, stirring frequently, until onions turn golden brown.
- Add garlic, chopped carrots, and spice mix to the pan. Cook and stir 1-1½ minutes, then remove from heat.
- When slightly cooled, add mix to blender or food processor and pulse 3-4x; add chickpeas and "eggs" and pulse 3-4x; push mix down then add breadcrumbs and pulse 5-6x until well blended but still slightly gritty.
- Oil fingertips and divide mix into 20 balls. Slightly flatten them into shape of your buns.
- Fry in small amount of oil until crisp and golden brown, then flip and repeat.

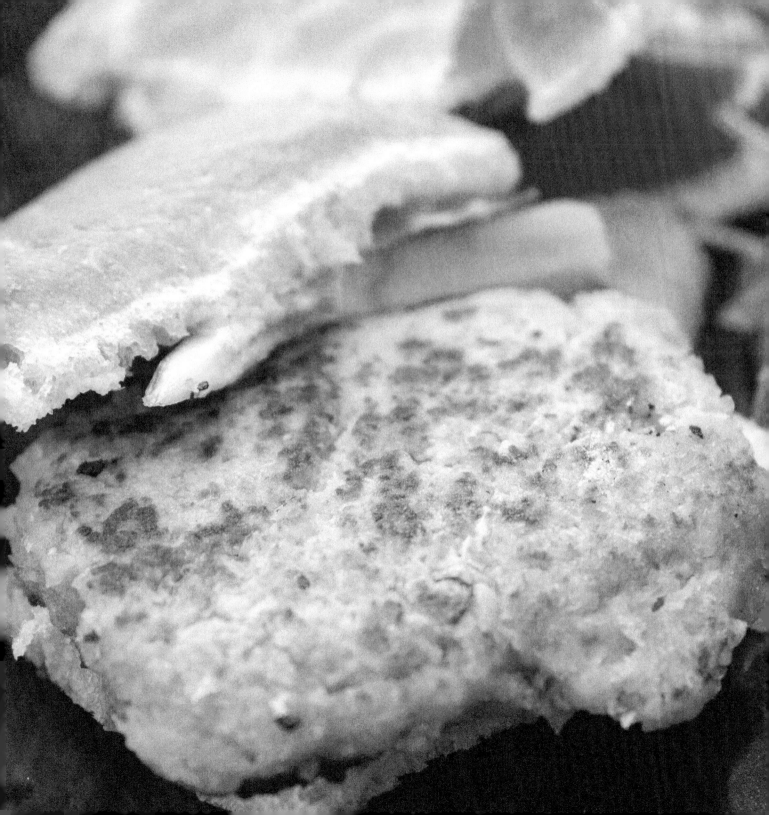

Appendix A: Replacing Animal Products with Plant Based Substitutes

If you're interested in revamping some of your favorite recipes to make them vegan, consider these substitutions.

Substitutions for eggs in baked goods include commercial products such as The Vegg® vegan egg yolk replacer, Ener-G egg replacer, Beyond Eggs, and The Neat Egg. Non-commercial substitutions include applesauce, a flax egg (one tablespoon ground flax seeds plus three tablespoons water blended), or mashed ripe banana. You'll have to experiment with your recipes to see what works best for you, provides the proper texture, and provides the best flavor.

For burgers, meatloaf, and recipes where eggs serve as a binding agent, try replacing raw eggs with quick cooking or rolled oats, potato starch, arrowroot or cornstarch, peanut or cashew butter, bread crumbs soaked in plant milk, chickpea flour, or the commercial products listed above.

Plain unsweetened soy, almond or coconut yogurt make a great substitute for sour cream toppings on tacos, baked potatoes, burritos or fruit desserts, in sauces, or baked into cakes and cookies.

Convenient substitutions for honey are agave or pure maple syrup, brown rice syrup, and light or dark molasses.

There are a variety of commercial plant milks available at your grocery store made from soy, rice, almonds, cashews, hemp, and coconut. Use the thicker, richer nut milks to make buttermilk for any recipe by adding 1 Tablespoon of vinegar or fresh lemon juice to a cup of nut milk. Stir, then let it sit for 5-10 minutes; you'll see the curdling.

Vegan substitutions for mayonnaise, butter, cheese, meats, and ice cream are also widely available at supermarkets and health food stores. Since good taste and texture are individual things, you'll just have to experiment until you find something that works for your palate.

There are also several recipes included in this book for vegan mock meats, but if you're short on time, picking up prepared seitan in the refrigerated or freezer section of your favorite grocery store is the easy solution.

Appendix B: Setting Up Your Vegan Kitchen

Next time you head to your local farmer's market, natural-foods store, or neighborhood grocery chain, take this handy list along as a guide for what to stock up on. If you haven't already done so, clear out spices over a year old, and foods which are not part of your new eating plan. Stock your freezer, spice rack, pantry, and refrigerator with the following items. It's not necessary that you go out and spend a fortune buying everything immediately, but having most of them on hand will provide options for preparing a wide variety of delicious, nutritious vegan meals without a trip to the grocery store.

Condiments
Extra-virgin olive oil
Coconut oil
Red wine vinegar
White wine vinegar
Apple cider vinegar
Balsamic vinegar
Reduced-sodium soy sauce or Bragg's Liquid Aminos (less sodium)
Hoisin sauce
Sweet chile sauce
Toasted sesame oil
Sriracha or other hot sauce
Dijon mustard
Vegan ketchup
Creole or spicy brown mustard
Sweet or dill pickle relish
Vegetarian mayonnaise

Seasonings
Kosher or pink sea salt
Seasoning salt
Smoked salt

Bay leaves
Black peppercorns and pepper grinder
White pepper
Herbs and spices, assorted dried (basil, parsley leaves, thyme leaves, sweet paprika, smoked paprika, cayenne, cumin, onion powder, garlic powder, oregano leaves, curry, turmeric, dried red pepper flakes, coriander)
Favorite salt-free, all-purpose seasoning (such as Spike seasoning)
Onions – dried flakes
Pure lemon and vanilla extracts
Not-chicken broth cubes
Vegetable broth cubes
Not-beef broth cubes

Dry Goods
Pasta (made from artichokes, brown rice, quinoa, amaranth, etc.)
Pearl barley (quick-cooking is fine)
Millet
Quinoa

Nutritional yeast flakes
Egg replacement powder (for baking)
Rice (brown, long-grain white, Jasmine or basmati)
Black beans
Lentils
Chickpeas
Arrowroot powder or cornstarch
Baking soda
Aluminum free baking powder
Chickpea flour
All purpose gluten free flour
Spelt or whole wheat flour (Look at the many options besides wheat. Store opened packages in the refrigerator or freezer in zip style bag)
Rolled or steel cut oats
Low fat granola
Whole grain crackers
Unsweetened cocoa powder

Nuts, Seeds & Fruits
(Store opened packages of nuts and seeds in the refrigerator or freezer for maximum freshness)
Raw walnuts
Raw almonds
Raw cashews
Natural peanut butter and/or other nut butter with no additives
Raw pumpkin seeds (pepitas), sesame seeds, sunflower seeds
Chia seeds
Tahini (sesame paste)

Dried apricots, cranberries, dates, and raisins

Canned, Cartoned & Bottled Goods
Sun dried tomatoes
Low sodium vegetable broth
"Not-chicken" vegetarian chicken-style broth
Mushroom broth
"Lite" coconut, almond or rice milk
Tomatoes: chopped, fire roasted and sauce
Tomato paste
Beans: black, kidney, pinto, Great Northern, cannellini, chickpeas

Refrigerator Items
Plant milk (nut, cashew, hemp, coconut or rice)
Vegan not-chicken seasoning paste
Corn or sprouted grain tortillas
Lettuce
Green beans
Pico de gallo or salsa
Carrots
Red bell peppers
Tofu (non-GMO, organic)
Tempeh
Celery
Vegan butter spread
Vegan cheese strips
Green onions
Kale
Collard greens

Spinach
Broccoli
Zucchini
Hummus (or make your own)
Cabbage
Leeks
Brussels sprouts
Cauliflower
Mushrooms

Frozen vegetables: peas and carrots,
chopped spinach, chopped broccoli, organic
corn, edamame
Veggie burger patties
Vegan sausage patties

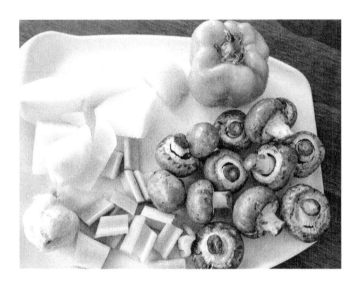

Pantry Items
Onions (red, white and yellow)
Garlic, fresh
Shallots, fresh
Avocados
Agave nectar (light) or pure maple syrup
Grape seed oil
Extra virgin olive oil
Vegan pasta sauce (in jars)
Ezekiel or other whole grain or sprouted
grain bread
Yams
Sweet potatoes
Pita bread
Hemp, pea or peanut protein powder
Organic apples, oranges, bananas, lemons,
grapefruit

Freezer
Frozen organic strawberries, blueberries,
mango, peaches
Buy fresh organic bananas, then peel and
freeze them in zip style bags

Appendix C: Guidelines for Daily Vegan Nutrition

What's listed below was approved for me by my personal physician and my dietitian as I transitioned to vegan, so I'm sharing with you. Notice the ranges given with regards to quantity of each food group. The precise item and amount of food you eat in each group will be determined by your activity level, age, and any health considerations you may have (like diabetes, heart disease, food allergies, etc.).

The total quantity of food you eat may also vary from day to day based on hunger. Hypertensives and adults over the age of 50 should pay special importance to sodium intake.

Always check with your doctor or a registered dietitian if you have any concerns about what to eat and your health.

Fruits (3-4 servings daily)

Fruit is the cleanser of the body and is usually an excellent source of Vitamin C and fiber. It is better to eat the whole fruit than it is to drink juice, as you get the benefits of fiber and other possibly unknown nutrients.

Strawberries, peaches, cherries, blackberries, oranges, blueberries, apples, bananas, pineapple, kiwi, cantaloupe, watermelon are excellent choices. Dried fruits like raisins, dates, cranberries, and mango are higher in calories, but great additions to breakfast cereal.

1 medium piece of fruit

½ cup canned or frozen fruit

½ large fruit

½ cup cooked fruit

¼ cup dried fruit

4 ounces fruit juice

Legumes (3-6 servings daily)

Includes beans, peas, chickpeas, lentils, and soy-based products (soy milk, tofu, tempeh, and textured vegetable protein)

½ cup cooked beans

½ cup (4 ounces) tofu or tempeh

8 ounces of soy milk

Nuts and Seeds (1-3 servings daily)

1 ounce (about ¼ cup) nuts, sunflower or pumpkin seeds

2 Tablespoons nut butter

3 Tablespoons chia seeds

Whole Grains (5-8 servings daily)

Corn, buckwheat, tortillas, bread, whole grain pasta, steel cut and rolled oats, brown and wild rice, grits, polenta, bread, pasta, millet, Cream of Wheat, etc.

1 cup cooked hot cereal

1 cup of ready-to-eat cereal

½ cup cooked brown rice, pasta, millet, etc.

1 slice of bread

¼ of a large bagel

½ a muffin

1 small pancake (6" round)

½ tortilla

½ pita

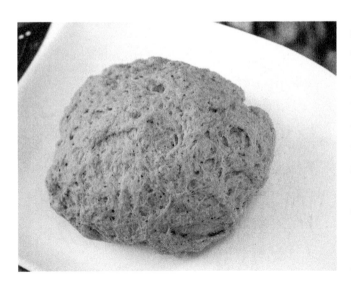

Vegetables (4-6 servings daily)

Emphasize dark green leafy vegetables for half your veggie intake. Collard, mustard and turnip greens, kale, bok choy, arugula, watercress, cabbage, broccoli and Brussels sprouts, as well as spinach and romaine lettuce all fall into this category.

Dark yellow and orange vegetables like yams, butternut squash, carrots, pumpkin, spaghetti squash, as well as zucchini, peppers, cucumbers and eggplant boost your daily fiber intake and supply a wide variety of vitamins and minerals.

1 cup raw vegetables

½ cup cooked vegetables

Herbs, Spices and Plant Oils (0-5 servings daily)

Herbs and spices — either fresh or dried — should be used liberally to add flavor interest to your food. Don't be afraid to experiment. Oils are high in calories, but add flavor. A small amount of oil can help spices "stick to" food, and prevent food from sticking to the pan. Use only as much as you need. Using water and oil to sauté prevents sticking and reduces the need for large amounts of oil. Make fried dishes no more than once per week.

1 teaspoon oil: coconut, olive, grape seed, sunflower or other plant or nut oil

Water

Though not usually considered part of "daily nutrition", my years as a fitness professional taught me that most people are dehydrated. They don't KNOW it, but their skin, urine color and slow hair growth shows that they are.

Researchers say our bodies are 60-70% water, and that we can live for weeks without food, but will die within days without water.

Web MD emphasizes the importance of water intake by stating: "Water keeps every part of your body working properly. It helps your body flush wastes and stay at the right temperature. It can help prevent kidney stones and constipation. You lose water throughout the day—through your breath, sweat, urine, and bowel movements. If you live in a hot climate, you lose even more fluid. You need to replace this lost fluid to stay healthy. If you don't get enough water, you could become dehydrated. If you get very dehydrated, your body no longer has enough fluid to get blood to your organs. This is dangerous."

If drinking water is difficult because you don't like plain water, try infusing your water with the essence of fruit.

Drop ¼ cup blueberries, ¼ cup halved strawberries, and ¼ cup raspberries into 2 cups of water (I use mason jars available by the dozen at mass retailers and grocery stores). Refrigerate for several hours, then enjoy.

Another tasty infused water uses citrus fruits. Slice an organic orange, lemon, and lime and put them in a mason jar. Fill to the top with filtered water. Screw on the top and refrigerate for several hours then enjoy.

Cucumbers and mint make a great infusion as well. Slice up ½ an organic cucumber and add it to your mason jar. Throw in about one-third cup of mint leaves (whatever your favorite is). Top with water and store away as above.

Drinking lemon water is a trick I learned from my grandmother, and I do it as often as possible. All you have to do is keep a pitcher of water at room temperature. The type with the built-in filtration system is perfect.

Every morning just pour a tall glass of water, and squeeze the juice of one whole lemon into it. Grandmother swore that it helped prevent illness and arthritis pain, cleared out mucus, freshened breath, and helped get the digestive tract moving to prevent constipation.

Some doctors tout lemon water as a weight loss and liver cleansing aid as well.

Appendix D: Plant based Sources of Four Vital Nutrients

Calcium, iron, protein and Vitamin D are important to the human body — brittle bones, osteoporosis, and anemia can result from insufficient intake of these vital minerals.

Though dairy products and meat are usually the "go to" source, all four nutrients listed above are available through fruits, vegetables, nuts and seeds.

Plant Based Sources of Iron

Iron is used to manufacture red blood cells, which carry oxygenated blood throughout the body. A deficiency in iron (anemia) may result in a pale complexion and lethargy. Iron requirements vary by gender, with males requiring 10 mg of iron per day, and females of childbearing years approximately 18 mg.

Heme-iron (the type of iron found in red meat and other animal products), is more readily absorbed by the body. However, of the iron found in meat, fish and poultry, only about 40% is heme iron — the other 60% is non-heme iron - the same as that found in grain products, fruits and vegetables, nuts, seeds, and legumes. You can easily meet your daily requirements for iron without utilizing animal sources.

Eating iron rich foods along with Vitamin C increases the absorption of iron into the bloodstream by as much as 400%. Taking advantage of this benefits achieved via this combination of foods is especially important for pregnant women, vegetarians, and vegans.

Iron Rich Grain Products

Oat and wheat bran, in addition to being excellent for lowering cholesterol, are also loaded with iron. A 3.5 oz serving of either Special K or Bran Wheat cereals will provide you with 13 mg of iron, just under 75% of your daily RDA.

Oatmeal and bulgur wheat both provide about 1.8 mg iron per cup, and Cream of Wheat brand cereal a whopping 10 mg per one cup serving.

One cup of cooked spaghetti (enriched) has approximately 2 mg of iron.

Beans, Nuts and Seeds

Soybeans and lentils are the clear winner here, with a one cup serving clocking 8.8 and 6.6 gms of iron, respectively. If you enjoy eating tofu, you'll be glad to know that each 4 ounce serving of firm tofu provides 6.4 mg of iron. Chickpeas and tempeh provide a respectable 4.5 gms per one cup serving.

Throw two tablespoons of tahini in with your chickpeas when you make hummus, and you'll boost the iron content by another 2.8 gms. Other beans like pinto, black, kidney, and black eyed peas are around 4.0 gms of iron per serving.

Nuts and seeds tend to be higher in calories, but are valuable sources of iron as well. A one cup serving of cooked quinoa provides 2.8 mg of iron. A one ounce serving of sunflower or pumpkin seeds, or one cup of soy milk provides 1.4 mg of iron.

One tablespoon of sesame seeds provides 1.2 mg of iron. A half-cup serving of canned Lima beans, kidney or garbanzo beans provides approximately 2 mg of iron.

Get Iron in Vegetables and Fruit

Eating vegetables such as one cup of cooked spinach (6.4 gms), turnips (3.2 gms), beet greens (2.7 gms), or collard greens (2.2 gms), provides fiber and lots of other vitamins and minerals.

A medium-sized baked potato is a good source of iron, providing about 2.5 mg per. Dried fruit has a significant amount of iron if you can handle the calorie hit. Four dried figs contain an impressive 3.4 mg of iron.

Try seedless raisins, or dried prunes, apricots, or peaches for around 1.5 mg of iron per ½ cup serving.

Cook in Cast Iron Pots

Turns out the advice to cook in cast iron cookware to increase your daily iron intake isn't an old wives tale after all. In a study published in 1986 in the Journal of the American Dietetic Association, researchers cooked 20 different foods in new cast iron skillets to test the iron absorption rate.

Findings state that iron levels increased in each item, with some more than quadrupling their iron content. For example, the iron in three ounces of applesauce increased from 0.35 mg to 7.3 mgs. Even eggs, already a reasonably high source of iron at 1.5 mg each, tripled their iron content to almost 4.76 mg.

Cooking acidic foods such as tomato based pasta sauces or soups proved to be an ideal way to increase iron absorption. A three ounce serving of pasta sauce showed an increase in iron content from 0.6 mg to 5.7 mgs.

Plant Based Sources of Protein

Protein is one of the three macro-nutrients (along with carbohydrates and fat), essential for human growth, development and health. Protein is necessary for muscle growth and repair after workouts as well.

How much protein do you need on a daily basis? The Harvard School of Public Health Institute of Medicine recommends that adults eat eight grams of protein per 20 pounds of body weight. Most Americans eat far too much protein.

Protein is useful in any weight loss program, as it has been proven to provide satiety and make it easier for dieters to stick to their programs. Choosing low fat protein sources reduces calorie intake and is a smarter choice for anyone attempting to lose weight.

Soy is a great source of protein, especially for vegans. Tempeh and cooked soybeans deliver a whopping 30 gms of protein per cup. A four oz serving of firm style tofu provides about 11 grams of protein. Many tofu manufacturers have begun to make low fat or "lite" versions of their products, which reduces fat content by 50 percent or more.

Seitan or "wheat meat" is very high in protein, providing about 21 gms of protein per three ounce serving.

When it comes to beans and bean products, this fiber rich, top quality low fat source of protein for vegans can't be beat. Lentils come in number one at 18 gms per serving with black beans, kidney beans, navy beans, great northern beans, black-eyed peas, pinto beans, chickpeas, lima beans and veggie burgers/dogs providing between 12-16 gms of protein per one cup serving.

Raw nuts and seeds provide less protein than beans, but add variety and important fats to the diet. Try adding ¼ cup of almonds (8 gms), sunflower seeds (6 gms), cashews (5 gms), or walnuts (4 gms) to your smoothies or salads.

Plant Based Sources of Calcium

Minerals, including calcium, are essential for good health. Calcium is the most abundant mineral in the body, comprising approximately two percent of your body's total weight.

Without the proper balance of minerals your muscles wouldn't contract, your heart would skip beats or stop beating altogether, your bones and teeth would become porous and soft, and your nervous system would not send the proper impulses to muscles and organs. Calcium is especially important for blood pressure regulation, utilization of insulin, blood clotting, and a strong skeletal system.

Though milk, cheese and other dairy products are marketed to be the primary sources for calcium, there are many other non-dairy products which provide high levels of usable calcium as well.

A diet which includes calcium rich foods from a variety of sources makes it much easier to meet daily calcium requirements.

Not sure how much calcium you should be aiming for? USDA 2010 Dietary Guidelines recommended daily requirements for calcium intake are:

700 mg per day for toddlers 1-3 years old
1000 mg per day for children 4-8 years of age
1300 mg per day for children and teens ages 9-18
1000 mg for adults 18-70
1200 mg per day for females 50+
1300 mg for 14-18 year old pregnant/lactating teens
1000 mg for 19-50 year old pregnant/lactating women

Non-Dairy Sources of Calcium

One cup of chopped cooked collard greens (previously frozen) provides 357 mg of calcium. Fresh cooked spinach (one cup) provides 245 mg, and a cup of cooked Black-eyed peas contains 211 mg of calcium.

One quarter cup (two ounces) of sesame seeds has 351 mg, one tablespoon of blackstrap molasses about 137 mg, and two cups of boiled broccoli 124 mg of calcium.

Almonds make a delicious energy producing snack, and offer 75 mg of calcium per one ounce serving. A big juicy orange or one quarter cup fresh boiled soybeans (edamame) each have about 55 mg of calcium.

Calcium Fortified Foods

Commercial food manufacturers frequently fortify breakfast cereals, tortillas, breads, muffins, and packaged juices with calcium. Total cereal from General Mills contains 258 mg of calcium per three quarter cup serving, and a six ounce serving of fortified orange juice about 220 mg.

Many non-dairy milk beverages made from rice and soy are also calcium enriched. Rice Dream is a popular choice for those allergic to both milk products and soy; its calcium enriched product offers approximately 130 mg of calcium per half cup serving.

Steroid medications decrease the body's ability to absorb calcium. If you are taking this type of medication, talk to your doctor about the possible need to add calcium supplements.

Plant Based Sources of Vitamin D

Be sure to make sure you're getting enough vitamin D as well, as it helps the body absorb calcium. If you don't get out in the sun much and aren't eating meat, you're likely to be deficient in this key vitamin which helps bones grow in children, and stay strong in adults.

Vitamin D deficiencies have been linked to several cancers (breast, colon cancer, and prostate), heart disease, depression, weight gain, and other afflictions.

Though there is no inarguable proof that a vitamin D deficiency causes these diseases, I prefer to err on the side of caution. Especially since people with more melanin in their skin need greater amounts of sun exposure to make vitamin D than those with lighter skin.

African-Americans living in the northern regions of the U.S. and in Canada should be aware of this possible problem, and its contribution to a vitamin D deficiency. Recommendations are for thirty minutes of sun exposure to the face, legs, or torso (without sunscreen), 2-3x per week.

Talk with your doctor to see if a supplement may be necessary. Aim for 600 IU per day with food and/or supplements.

Enriched soy products, fortified almond milk, ready-to-eat breakfast cereals, fortified orange juice, portobello and maitake mushrooms are all great sources of vitamin D for vegans.

Appendix E: The Most and Least Pesticide Laden Fruits and Vegetables

The Environmental Working Group (EWG) prepares an annual report which identifies the most pesticide-laden fruits and vegetables sold in the U.S. Scientists working with EWG focus on 48 of the most popular produce items, and develop rankings based on an analysis of more than 30,000 samples tested by the USDA and the FDA. Based on the 2014 report, it is strongly suggested that we purchase organic versions of "the Dirty Dozen" (the top 12 most pesticide laden fruits and vegetables), to avoid exposure to these heavily sprayed items. Some people say they don't believe in buying organic foods, or that they're too expensive. Budget considerations are certainly important, but so is the long-term health of you and your family.

A 2012 report by the American Academy of Pediatrics pointed out that children are more likely to be impacted by heavy doses of pesticides, which could cause learning disorders and pediatric cancers. Residue of chemical contaminants including DDT (banned in the US since the 1970s, but still used in other countries), have been found in blood, urine and even breast milk. Researchers at Rutgers University have linked DDT exposure to late-onset Alzheimer's Disease. Other studies show links to diseases and illnesses such as birth defects, asthma, diabetes, various forms of cancer, rheumatoid arthritis, and Parkinson's disease. Buying organic when you can just makes sense. Find out more at www.beyondpesticides.org.

The 16 Most Pesticide Laden Foods (non-organic)

1. apples
2. strawberries
3. grapes
4. celery
5. peaches
6. spinach
7. sweet bell peppers
8. nectarines (imported)
9. cucumbers
10. cherry tomatoes
11. snap peas (imported)
12. potatoes
13. hot peppers
14. blueberries (domestic)
15. lettuce
16. kale/collard greens

The Sweet 16 (least pesticide-laden)

1. avocados
2. sweet corn
3. pineapples
4. cabbage
5. sweet peas – frozen
6. onions
7. asparagus
8. mangoes
9. papayas
10. kiwi fruit
11. eggplant
12. grapefruit
13. cantaloupe
14. cauliflower
15. sweet potatoes
16. mushrooms

Carrots came in at #22, green beans at #24, and broccoli at #28 on the list. Tomatoes were #33, mushrooms #26, and bananas #32.

Appendix F: Equivalent Measurements

This	Equals This
3 teaspoons	1 Tablespoon
4 Tablespoons	¼ cup
5⅓ Tablespoons	⅓ cup
8 Tablespoons	½ cup
16 Tablespoons	1 cup
2 Tablespoons (liquid)	1 ounce
1 cup	8 fluid ounces
2 cups	1 pint / 16 fluid ounces
4 cups	1 quart
4 quarts	1 gallon
⅛ cup	2 Tablespoons
⅓ cup	5 Tablespoons + 1 teaspoon
⅔ cup	10 Tablespoons + 2 teaspoons
¾ cup	12 Tablespoons
1 pound butter	2 cups butter or margarine
1 stick butter	½ cup butter or margarine
1 lb box powdered sugar	3¾ cups powdered sugar

Recipe Index

Appetizers & Snacks

Breakfast Ideas

Desserts and Sweets

Entrées/Main Dishes

How To...

Smoothies

Acknowledgements

I wish to acknowledge the support, prodding (to hurry up and finish!), and cheer leading I received on this project from family and friends – both online and off. You happily volunteered to be guinea pigs for my concoctions, testing both foods I prepared and recipes in your own kitchens. Thankfully, not one of you got sick or died!

Shouts out to my parents who have been there since the beginning – literally. And to my brothers, you guys are the greatest brothers a sister could wish for. But don't think I've forgiven you for the time you took both hands to help your face chew the first pot roast I made because it was so tough.

Special thanks go to my aunts, uncles, grandmothers, my Mom, and all the men and women who let me into their kitchens over the years. Especially my Uncle Bill who took the time to show me how a few creative twists to plain home cooking can give any dish a real "professional chef" appearance and taste. From each of you I learned so much about cooking as a labor of love. And though all of you may not be around to read these words, I'm convinced you approve.

And the most heartfelt thank yous to Patricia and David, Joy and Don, Shelia, Anthony, and Gaynelle for being my biggest supporters. You wonderful people provided me with the things I needed to be successful, and showered me the kind of "got your back" love and encouragement that most people can only dream about.

CPSIA information can be obtained at www.ICGtesting.com
Printed in the USA
BVOW07s1709031115

425434BV00025B/171/P